UNWANTED BAGGAGE

Elizabeth Prosser
&
Philip Prosser

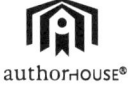

AuthorHouse™ UK Ltd.
500 Avebury Boulevard
Central Milton Keynes, MK9 2BE
www.authorhouse.co.uk
Phone: 08001974150

© 2011. Elizabeth Prosser & Philip Prosser. All rights reserved

No part of this book may be reproduced, stored in
a retrieval system, or transmitted by any means
without the written permission of the author.

First published by AuthorHouse 1/29/2011

ISBN: 978-1-4567-7155-3

This book is printed on acid-free paper.

Because of the dynamic nature of the Internet, any Web addresses or
links contained in this book may have changed since publication and
may no longer be valid. The views expressed in this work are solely those
of the author and do not necessarily reflect the views of the publisher,
and the publisher hereby disclaims any responsibility for them.

ACKNOWLEDGEMENTS

I would like to thank my husband Philip for his infinite patience, love, his help and his own contributions. Without his encouragement, I would never have written this book.

I would also like to mention my incredible Gastroenterologist, Dr. Russell Canavan, Surgeon, Mr David Jackson and my wonderful stoma nurses Mary Platt and Dwynwyn; all the staff at Bronglais hospital, specifically, those on Meurig & ICU Wards. My GP's, Dr James (now retired), Dr James (new to the practice), Dr Thomas, Dr Langley and all the staff at Tregaron Surgery who have been incredibly caring and patient. Without these good people, I probably would not be here to tell the tale.

Thanks to my beautiful daughter Tamara, whose constant transatlantic encouragement and love has helped me to complete this work so that it will aid in the healing process.

Credit is also due to both my dear mother, Betty Lloyd, and the best mother-in-law in the world, Ruth Prosser for their ongoing support and love.

I would also like especially to thank my stepson, Andrew Prosser, who has always been there for us. He is a devoted and much loved progeny who I regard as my own. He has a good understanding of my illness and even helped by creating all the cartoons herein.

I must add my dearest cousin Meriel, who, throughout my life has always been closer than any sister could have been. She will never know how much her support and love has meant to me.

True friends are hard to come by – but I have some special ones: my favourite bridesmaid, Sue, who has traipsed to the wilds of West Wales (once almost driving off the side of a mountain), on many occasions to raise my spirits, often dragging our good pal Caroline in her wake! I must also mention all the class of SHS '69, especially Louise, Julia, Deborah, Judy, Helen, Janice, and Vanessa – I look forward to our 60th reunion! Recognition is due to one of my closest friends and neighbour Denise Hicks. Denise and her husband Geoff, together with our good friends, Richard and Jenny, went out of their way to make us welcome when we moved to our village.

Thanks especially to all the local **CROHN'S AND COLITIS UK** organizing team, especially Chris and Mike (you now who you are!), not only for their support but also for their friendship and handholding. They have always been on the other end of a phone for both of us.

Last, but not least, I must also mention Pelican Healthcare and Bullen Healthcare, two manufacturers who have made my ostomy life comfortable. In particular, Julie St John from Pelican for her support of our local newsletter and their wonderful product range and Sharon Levy, my friendly Bullen representative for her advice and sense of humour, especially when it comes to bag covers! Thanks also to Jeremy Eakin (Eakin Group), who came to my rescue after an extremely difficult leakage problem.

INTRODUCTION

Why did I write this book? Faced with having to carry around my unwanted baggage with me for the rest of my life, I knew it would be therapeutic to share my experiences with my fellow ostomates. I must stress that I am not a medical professional. The information contained in this book is based solely on my own unbiased personal research and experience. If you are visiting a new country, you may consult a guidebook – This is your guidebook to the Ostomy World.

As a new ostomate, I ransacked the internet and libraries for every scrap of information on ostomies. Whilst there was little current information in the published domain, I found many websites all giving conflicting, or complicated explanations and suggestions. However, apart from some of the ostomy blog sites, very little of this was provided by ostomates themselves or written from a personal perspective or experience.

Individual manufacturers are obviously interested in promoting their own products. Larger manufacturers sponsor stoma nurses in some National Health Trusts and use this influence to prioritise their products. This naturally gives an unhelpful start to many stoma patients who are misled into believing that they have no choice other than to use the hospital's recommended service or manufacturer. You are of course, free to choose and sample any number of products during the lifetime of your ostomy.

Medical and amateur "specialists" advise on the best way to choose and cope with ostomy bags - without ever having worn one! One classic example of advice, found on several websites, tells patients that the best way to empty a bag is to sit on the toilet and empty the bag between the legs. As anyone who has ever tried this will tell you – this will end in disaster, with splashes galore and a general inability to clean the bag's open end properly!!! Be warned, a model can do this in a picture with an empty bag but it is nearly impossible in reality.

People who have not experienced an ostomy cannot possibly imagine the reality of life-changing surgery, waking up to a stoma and learning to live with all the complications it brings. I decided to put together almost everything that you might need to know after having, or be about to have, ostomical surgery. I wanted to create a book containing everything I could think of to help people find answers, comfort and help - all the things that my family gave me. I now consider myself to be an *"expert ostomy patient"* * and as such, will help you through the minefield of products and services that you will meet on your ostomical voyage.

Note: The NHS currently runs an excellent **Expert Patients Programme, to encourage people to understand their individual chronic illness, in order that they can learn, maintain and cope with all aspects of their condition. The aim of this programme is to reduce the number of times a patient will have to call upon NHS professionals over minor issues but also to know when they should seek professional assistance.*

People have ostomies caused by bowel and urinary diseases, cancers, related accidental damage and birth defects. Major additional research is desperately needed into the causes and treatments that might prevent future ostomies. A stoma is a lifelong, permanent appendage as much as a nose or an ear, – and, as with other appendages, things can go wrong occasionally. Additional research is also required into the field of post surgical stoma complications.

CROHN'S AND COLITIS UK (formerly NACC) is the largest organisation contributing to research into the medical, social and psychological aspects of IBD (inflammatory bowel disease). It supports stem cell research as it applies to IBD. They also continue to put pressure on **NICE** (the National Institute for Clinical Excellence) for the introduction of related new medications into the NHS. For the latest information on progress made through NICE, the website address is:

www.nice.org.uk

CROHN'S AND COLITIS UK is a wonderful hands-on organisation. They do not waste their money on massive directors' salaries or glamorous office space. They work in cramped surroundings with many volunteers. **CROHN'S AND COLITIS UK** brings together people of all ages who have Crohn's Disease or Ulcerative Colitis, which includes Proctitis. It extends help and information (and even financial support in some cases), to the families, carers and health professionals.

CROHN'S AND COLITIS UK was there for me from the time I was diagnosed with Crohn's disease. I joined the local CROHN'S AND COLITIS UK group that has not only given me a great deal of support, but also introduced me to a new circle of friends and fellow patients. I cannot speak highly enough of this network and encourage fellow ostomates to seek out similar, relevant groups:

- **The Colostomy Association**

    www.colostomyassociation.org.uk

- **The Ileostomy and Internal Pouch Support Group www.the-ia.org.uk**

- **Crohn's and Colitis UK (Formerly the National Association for Colitis and Crohn's disease)**

- **The Urostomy Association of Great Britain www.uagbi.org.uk**

Notes on the use of the term "Disabled"

You will notice many references to ***"disabled".*** You may think this excludes you. However, in your interests, it does not! Please read on....

No one likes to think of themselves as less abled, but the term itself is not a stigma; on the contrary, having a stoma gives you entitlements and benefits that help make life a little easier. In addition, many stoma patients have other illnesses or difficulties that make mobility a problem. Others simply need the use of an accessible, 'disabled' toilet, equipped with a sink and shelf to change and empty their bags.

There are times when the illness that caused you to have a stoma leaves you weak and exhausted. Most medications that stoma patients are prescribed have side effects. Side effects may also contribute to physical and mental difficulties. All these conditions may make us less able to cope.

The Department of Works and Pensions (DWP) recognises that stoma patients qualify for a degree of **Disability Living Allowance (DLA)**, even if you are in full time employment.

Incapacity Benefit is also available to ostomates if you have been in employment and are no longer able to work due to related illness; the affects of surgery; medication, physical complications; mental stress or other psychological problems related to being an ostomate.

One of the single major benefits to this 'disabled' tag gives you the right to use a **disabled parking bay** (by means of a council supplied "**Blue Badge**"), nearest to accessible public toilets, and all the locations where they can also be found: - e.g. supermarkets, motorway service stations and airports. Details of these and many, many other benefits are included in the book in detail.

The railways' authorities include ostomates in their qualification for a '**Disabled Railcard'**.

Utility companies will give discounts, – in particular, water companies make quite considerable discounts for water and sewerage rates to ostomates, capping the annual bills, regardless of usage.

Labels are words. The tag 'disabled' covers a multitude of difficulties that people endure. Benefits accorded to ostomates do not make you feel better but they certainly make life easier. They are a small consideration to your ostomy and its needs. In no way should it be reflected as belittling, pitying or demeaning. A healthy ostomate always gets funny looks as they open the door to a disabled toilet, but trying to evacuate or change a bag is difficult in a standard toilet! Just put up with the looks or answer the unspoken questions. You are entitled to use these conveniences! Ignorance of the general public is no excuse to try to manage in an inconvenient setting.

"Time heals almost everything, give time, time!"

Purple ribbons are worn to show support for Fibromyalgia, Chronic Pain, Crohn's Disease, Lupus and Cystic Fibrosis.

Illustrations by Andrew Prosser
Crohn's Image by Grea

Graphic resolution images
by Ocula Photo, Aberystwyth

Contents

Chapter One
My Ostomical Story
...Another of life's adventures.
....1

Chapter Two
Ostomy Surgery
...An Introduction to the whys and wherefores.
....10

Chapter Three
Specific Symptoms and Treatments
...Finding a Diagnosis
....22

Chapter Four
If Surgery Is Necessary
...From Hospital Admittance to Discharge
....56

Chapter Five
The Stoma Nurse
...Meeting Your New Best Friend
....72

Chapter Six
Early Days
...The Beginning of Life after Surgery.
....75

Chapter Seven
Problem Areas
...How to recognise and deal with potential problems quickly.

....*87*

Chapter Eight
Hints and Tips
...A Few Ideas and Suggestions to Assist New Ostomates

....*107*

Chapter Nine
Irrigation
...A Viable Alternative?

....*111*

Chapter Ten
A Reversal
...Ostomy Reversal following temporary keyhole surgery.

....*116*

Chapter Eleven
A Post Operative Diet Guide
...Diet Guidance for Ostomy Patients

....*120*

Chapter Twelve
Exercise & Sports
...Guidelines for Activities
....*138*

Chapter Thirteen
Travelling with a stoma
...Hints and Tips for UK and International Adventures
....*152*

Chapter Fourteen
Appliances and Accessories
...All the essentials on bags and necessary extras
....*219*

Chapter Fifteen
Benefits and Entitlements
.. Chronic Illness can bring Financial problems in its wake: Central, local government and other sources can help.
....*271*

Chapter Sixteen
Emotions
Emotional adjustment to life with a chronic Illness
....*295*

**Chapter Seventeen
Intimacy**
.. Up close and personal
..301

**Chapter Eighteen
Children and Young People**
... the world of young ostomates
..316

**Chapter Nineteen
Ostomical Workplace**
... Returning to, or starting work with an ostomy
..353

**Chapter Twenty
Leaving work**
... Retiring, ill health, or to become a full or part-time carer
..368

**Chapter Twenty One
Pregnancy and Childbirth**
... Yes, you Can!
..375

**Chapter Twenty two
Caring**
... Life as a Carer
..381

Chapter Twenty-three
Cooking for Carers
... Strangers to the kitchen?
....*399*

The Website
...The Future World of Unwanted baggage
....*410*

Everything Else
websites and other useful information
....*412*

Chapter One
My Ostomical Story
...Another of life's adventures.

Until my early fifties, I enjoyed a lifetime of reasonably good health. However, without warning, I collapsed in March 2004. I was rushed to hospital with a mystery illness and a subsequent diagnosis of fibromyalgia was pronounced. It then took many, many tests and several years before a diagnosis of Crohn's was added. Due to complications with medication, I also developed epilepsy, and, after a bout of shingles, I was left with post herpetic neuralgia (I never do things by half!).

With Crohn's, came many new interests in life: I developed an unhealthy interest in the location of public toilets. I discovered an atlas of the UK showing every public loo and even a Sat. Nav. lavatory finder!

I began to give directions to other people using loos instead of pubs! My shopping cart overflowed with different brands of toilet paper to test run them for softness, absorption and grab-ability! I cannot say who the winner is, but the puppy is cute. On one occasion, at the till, I was rushed to the staff toilet by an ashen-faced checkout girl; until I realised that I had mistakenly produced my "***Can't Wait***" card instead of my Visa card!

> The holder of this card has a medical condition and needs to use toilet facilities
>
> # URGENTLY!

Instead of outings to shopping Malls, I began to have excursions to hospitals. I met so many new people - gastroenterologists, radiologists, phlebotomists, pain specialists, anaesthetists, neurologists, physiotherapists, colorectal surgeons, stoma nurses, maxillofacial surgeons all of whom conversed in a special medical language that, when written resembled hieroglyphics to the lay-patient.

I needed a GPS system to find a new wealth of departments I never new existed within the sacred clinic walls. I soon discovered that it was really necessary to *"say yes"* to sedation when examinations consisted of optic cameras being inserted into places where photography is not normally an issue. I even began to collect more photos of my insides than I had of my outsides. I even had a favourite arm for Intravenous infusions.

Hospital staff working in the gastroenterology departments have a wicked sense of humour! The colour and consistency of poo is a constant topic. They even have pictures and charts of it all over the walls. When the world drops out of your bottom rather than the other way round, they maintain a calm dignity in taking care of your predicament.

Unwanted Baggage

When I visited friends, they asked after my bowels before my family, and I was shown the loo before being offered tea and biscuits. I am convinced that my friends began to have their suspicions about my habits when they viewed my bruised arms and veins and saw the contents of my handbag, stuffed with pills and vials of all descriptions among the debris of used tissues, keys and make-up.

Things began to get difficult when I realised I would have to invoke the lesser-known 'slave' clause in the marriage vows. I found it increasingly difficult to stay upright. I was prescribed so much pain medication that I fell asleep on my feet when I did manage to stand. Luckily, my other half bravely donned a pinny and set about disproving the myth that men cannot multi-task.

Nevertheless, just as I thought things could not get any worse, I was rushed into hospital for emergency surgery. Diagrams were produced and I heard words like "sub-total colectomy", "ileostomy", "bowel removal" and nodded sagely; but apart from trying to ask sensible questions (like asking the surgeon to remove some unsightly fat while he was in there), I did not absorb the real implications.

I woke up after a good six-hour, drug induced nap to emerge into the new world of ICU – I felt like a bionic woman with tubes going every which way, connected to a variety of machines competing tunefully with each other. It was Christmas Eve, and the staff thoughtfully believed we would enjoy the benefits of the season. Normally I am the first one to put the CDs on, with Bing Crosby singing while I make Christmas cakes! Lying in a hospital bed following major surgery, in a drug induced haze - lets just say I did not find "God rest ye merry gentlemen" sung loudly by a group of enthusiastic visiting carollers, to be the most appropriate welcome back to the real world.

Other than that, I do not remember my first few days until I was moved to a high dependency unit where the staff remained ever vigilant. Fortunately, through these first few dark times, visiting was unlimited for family. My husband spent so much time in hospital that he thought he had earned the right to wear a white coat and join the doctor's rounds.

The nursing team gave me a magic button to administer pain medication all by myself. That was the first sign that I was not going to be too pleased when I really surfaced from my post-operative, drug induced state. However, after a few days I knew I would have to grin and bare all. After all the tubes and drips were removed, I realised one item was permanent. I had acquired a new appendage.

When they said, "You've got a bag!" I thought "Well, better than flowers; a colourful Gucci perhaps? Perchance a Burberry"? Alas, it was a neutral beige and, rather than carrying it around in my hand, it was attached to my abdomen in such a way that I realised it was there to stay. I had a "stoma", an opening from the colon to the surface of the abdomen to deliver waste.

Before the "Grand Opening", I was introduced to my newly appointed "Best Friend". I was just about to explain that, despite appearances to the contrary, I actually had quite a lot of friends, when Mary Platt came into my life (aka "Angel of the Stoma World"). Mary, my personal stoma nurse (we all get one!), came into my life at a time when I felt I was down so far, I felt I would never again see the daylight from

Unwanted Baggage

the 'Slough of Despond' I had sunk into. (Apologies to John Bunyan, but Christian never had an ileostomy).

Mary explained that she was my Stoma Nurse and she kept me amused with tall tales of ostomy adventures. She soon got down to the nitty-gritty and, locating my husband reading the five-year-old magazines in the ward's day room, we began our conference 'a trois'. She explained that the philosophy of having fathers in attendance at the birth of their child also applied to the introduction of partners to stomas. I am sure that there are many who eagerly await the results of their partner's surgery – new, bigger breasts! Flat tummies, thin thighs…but believe me, this is *NOT* the same. Initially the nurses were excellent at keeping things covered and me in the dark. To be honest I was quite terrified at what might be revealed under all the gauze and how my husband would react.

As she shredded gauze, applied lotions and revealed all, I saw that where my smooth stomach had been (OK, after 4 children there were a few wrinkles and the surgeon had not taken the wonderful opportunity to remove the teensy minor, quite large, amount of excess fat), there was now a mouth-like opening which seemed to be oozing slightly. She asked me if I felt ready to clean the area. We both anxiously watched my husband. He jumped in, offered to take on the task, and, under her supervision washed the area, and managed to fit a new bag in the right place. He did not seem in the least perturbed and Mary gave him a ten out of ten. I got a measly three for my subsequent try – my claim is that while they were looking down, I was lying flat trying to effectively *"pin the tail on the donkey"* without the benefit of facing it!

Through her help, all embarrassment between us dissolved and she began to chat about her future role in our lives. She told me that she would visit when I was discharged; be there when I needed her; in person or on the other end of a phone or email. She explained that she was there to help with everything not only the physical side of ostomy problems but also to alleviate and explain the emotional highs and lows that always accompany stoma patients. She explained that we would be "going shopping" for the ideal bag and all the other accessories needed to go with it. She undertook to order all the supplies I needed until I felt well enough to take the reins and with that, she wrote her number in indelible marker in a convenient place (don't ask!), and vanished into the mist from whence she had come.

After I was discharged, Mary was faithful to her word and arrived the next day, bringing boxes upon boxes of bags by different manufacturers. Her first home visit lasted three hours and six cups of tea! She did not hesitate to visit at any time I had problems always alerting us in advance to ensure that refreshments were ready.

After the first few weeks, I began to take interest in myself again. I looked a mess. My hair began to fall out and had gone white (apparently quite normal for major surgery – they do not tell you the good bits!), but eventually grew in again thicker and curlier than before. I found a good hair dye (essential, never, ever grow grey, gracefully). I applied make-up and perfume. I found that shopping (online of course), was my next essential as none of my clothing with a waistband fitted comfortably. (Any excuse will do for a new wardrobe!) I looked at specialised stoma clothing and underwear, high waist trousers and harem pants; decided

Unwanted Baggage

on a mix of yoga pants for indoor use and loose flowing dresses to receive visitors. French knickers became the order of the day and a whole new look emerged.

On a serious note, I was however, preoccupied with "me". I was and am undeniably very ill, but I initially acted as if I was the only person in the world with a stoma. I was angry at the way I looked; the scars that covered my entire abdomen, and the fact that I had to wear a bag for the rest of my life. I took that anger out on those who were going beyond to help me, especially my husband. Sometimes his total understanding of my emotional roller coaster only exacerbated my feelings. I must emphasise that every ostomy patient is different in their physical recovery and any pre-existing illness that may contribute to this recovery. In my own case, my lack of mobility due to my other illnesses added to my frustration. A stroke during my operation had also taken the sight of one eye - an unusual, added complication. I felt so helpless because I could not do things. I disliked having to dress for the bag and wear cover-up nightwear to hide my scars and bag. I believed my husband could no longer find me attractive; that my friends and family would think I was a burden to him and a nuisance to them.

Logically I knew this to be totally untrue but it took months of Phil's patience and love to bring me back to earth. Now, when leaky bags mean changing sheets and showering in the middle of the night, we find it an excuse for a late-night cuddle. The care and understanding that all my family and friends continue to show to me makes me realise that I am very lucky.

Without the life-saving, emergency surgery that I had, I would not be alive. Unfortunately, Crohn's is a disease that is subject to flare-ups and remissions. Since my surgery, I have had five serious physical flare-ups resulting in more hospital stays and another major operation to re-site the stoma.

As with any life-changing surgery, unwanted "bag"-gage takes a lot of adjustment emotionally as well as physically. I have read the blogs on "Crohn's zone" – everyone has emotional problems of one kind and another and we all deal with them differently as they arise. Even a young male ostomate admitted to "having a bit of a cry now and then". One thing we all seem to have in common is that silly things seem to upset us much more than problems with our illnesses or the associated physical issues.

Phil, as chief cook and bottle washer also continues to improve his skills, even proving that his Yorkshire pudding always rises perfectly. (Mine never did!) Despite growing our own vegetables, caring for our chickens pigs and calves, he continues to hone his domestic skills but he always, always has time for me.

If you feel like an invalid, you will continue to be one. I make every effort to appear as well as I can and take advantage of every opportunity to enjoy what I can – a good book, my laptop (or, as I think of it, my gateway to the outside world), a television programme, fresh flowers, anything that I find uplifting. I talk to my husband about how I feel and despite it adding to his concerns; it helps him to know I am able to talk about why I feel low.

The right kind of communication has become far more essential between us. Carers play a vital role in an ostomate's life but their lives change as much as their patient's does

Chapter Two
Ostomy Surgery
...An Introduction to the whys and wherefores.

People have always suffered with problems and diseases of the abdomen, bladder, bowel, intestines, and rectum. Surgical remedies have evolved to remove the affected parts. If those organs are removed in their entirety, the surgeon will create an ***Ostomy,*** or an artificial opening on the abdominal wall, using healthy tissue. The actual opening is called is a ***stoma***. When you look at the stoma, you are actually looking at the lining of the internal organ, exposed to the outside. It is warm and moist and secretes mucus. The stoma becomes an outlet for stomach waste or urine.

History

There is an early medical record on an Egyptian papyrus recommending honey as a dietary curative for abdominal complaints. Hieroglyphs show that surgeons learned processes to remove infected or enlarged organs – including the bowel - their research was due in part to the extensive embalming techniques and dissections allowed under ancient Egyptian religion,.

Unwanted Baggage

A fully recorded account of abdominal surgery is of an ostomy performed in 400 BC by the roman surgeon, Praxagore, His description leads us to think it was a colostomy – unfortunately, he did not tell how long his patient survived.

There follows many early records from various parts of the world, but detailed accounts are inexact until the eighteenth century. In 1706, a written account tells us of a colostomy performed in France by an unknown surgeon on a certain Georges Deppes, wounded at the battle of Ramiles. Apparently, Georges lived for a further fourteen years after his operation. Sixty years later, there is another tale of another French surgeon, Monsieur Pilore, performing a colostomy that allowed for a primitive collection apparatus comprised of a sponge attached to the body with an elastic bandage to the body.

From 1780-1900, colostomy operations continued to be performed successfully in France, by surgeons Messieurs Dupuytren and Maydl; in Germany, by Herren Mikulicz and Von Radecki; and in England by Messers Miles and Bryant.

Throughout the decades, faecal matter from the stoma drained into all manner of leather, glass and wooden receptacles. However, a drainable rubber bag system was not invented until World War II when, due to the amount of wound surgery to the abdomen, its need became more evident.

Urology surgery also has its roots documented on Egyptian papyrus. In addition, the mummified body of a 5,000 yr old child was discovered and found to contain a bladder that had been surgically altered. Obviously, surgery was unsuccessful but it serves an indication that bladder surgery was an early medical procedure. However, urology as a specialty in its own right was only instituted in 1890 with the appointment of Felix Guyon in Paris as the first French Professor of Urology.

No history of the development of urology is complete without mention of the contribution made by equipment companies. The mainstay of urology has always been telescopic examination of the urinary tract that until the 1950s was very basic. Early attempts at transmitting light down rigid telescopes were nothing if not innovative, ranging from candles to battery-driven lamps, but were fraught with the dual problems of clarity & reliability.

The crucial breakthrough, in the mid-1950s, was the development of the Hopkins® rod lens system. This revolutionized urology by providing robust, versatile, reliable & sterilisable endoscopic equipment and "cold" light sources that allowed high-quality visualization of the interior of the urinary tract. The later addition of fibre optic (flexible) endoscopes and endoscopic video cameras further enhanced operative urology. Such equipment was instrumental in the establishment of urology as a bona fide specialty in the 20th century. Urostomies lagged behind abdominal ostomies and it was not until the 1950s that the modern 'ileal conduits' or urostomies became standard procedures.

In 2010, patients have a tremendous choice in bags and pouches that make life easier for the ostomate (a patient who has undergone ostomy surgery).

Unwanted Baggage

Today, in many poorer countries where life-saving surgery is performed, there is little provision for aftercare or even for the basic essential collection of faeces or urine. Post-operative patients are discharged with rubber gloves, carrier bags and adapted coffee cans to act as faecal and urine receptacles. As the NHS, bag manufacturers and suppliers do not accept the return of any opened or part boxes of unused bags that you may have, you can now send bags and any unwanted accessories to the following charities, a wonderful way of recycling. Details of these are as follows:

Jacobs's Well appeal

Jacob's Well is a charity that supplies humanitarian aid to Eastern Europe and Asia. They will ensure that all medical supplies including stoma materials are sent to their depots in these countries.

To save postage costs remove any excess packaging – boxes and plastic packs just parcel up the bags and any associated wipes etc and send to:

Jacobs Well Appeal
2 Ladygate
Beverley
East Yorkshire HU17 8BH
Email: thejacobswell@aol.com

SCAR

(Stoma care and recovery) is a support group for overseas patients recovering from stomas. They supply many African countries, especially Uganda. Parcels can be sent to:

SCAR - Maggie Littlejohn
1B Redburg Gate
Kilwinning Road
Irvine KA12 8TH
Email maggielittlejohn@aol.com
www.fowusa.org/newsite

The Friends of Ostomates Worldwide-USA is a volunteer-run, non-profit organization providing ostomy supplies and educational materials to ostomates in need around the world.

All excess materials can be sent to the above address where a worldwide distribution network to supply needy ostomates is in place. They are urgently seeking paediatric ostomy and urostomy bags.

FOW-USA
1500 Arlington Avenue
Louisville, KY 40206-3177
USA

Unwanted Baggage

You now you've got IBD when……

- You have a favourite Ensure flavour.
- People ask about your guts, before they ask about your family.
- Most of your shopping trolley is toilet paper.
- You rattle because you take so many tablets
- You have more scars and bruises on your arm from blood tests, central lines and drains than a junkie!
- You have more photos of your insides that the outsides.
- Have a favourite arm for I.V's.
- Know that wearing white could be a <u>really big</u> mistake!
- You always have a spare pair of underwear in your bag/pocket.
- When you go on business visits, your clients offer you the toilet before the tea.
- You are not embarrassed about discussing <u>poo</u> anymore.
- The world falls out of your bottom, rather than the other way round.

- You give directions via toilets rather than by pubs.

- You start to look like a dealer with all the medication you carry around.

- You can take one look at your CAT scan and know if there is a problem!

- Your friends and family know how things are by looking at your plate.

- When everyone thinks your lovely bright pink cheeks are you being healthy, except of course you're at death's door and full to the brim with steroids.

- When you approach traffic lights and pray: "Please stay green, please stay green, <u>pleeeaaaasse</u>".

- The thing you get most excited about, when viewing new houses, is the size of the bathroom, and the strength of the flush on the toilet.

- At the checkout, you are surprisingly ushered to a toilet by an ashen-faced shop assistant with lightening speed, after mistaking your "Can't Wait" card for your VISA card!

The Ostomy situation in the UK today

If a patient does not respond well to other treatment, ostomies are performed. They are the last line of defence in the following illnesses or conditions:

- Crohn's disease
- Ulcerative colitis
- Colorectal cancer
- Diverticular disease
- Accidental damage to the bowel
- Congenital defects

To date, figures are only kept in individual hospitals, so accuracy is difficult to achieve. However, based on telephone surveys to some Health Trusts, at least 750,000 people in the UK have been recorded as having a permanent ostomy. Permanent ostomical surgery is a life-changing operation after which a patient will live a reasonably normal life with the addition of an ostomy bag, but in most cases, without the severe abdominal pain caused by the disease that necessitated the operation in the first place. In some cases, a temporary colostomy is performed through keyhole surgery. This allows to the colon to rest and recover for about six months after which another keyhole operation (a reversal) is required. Unfortunately, many reversal operations also fail after several years resulting in permanent surgery.

Stomas are sited on the wall of the abdomen so that they can be easily reached for changing and cleaning. With a colostomy or ileostomy, a special bag (or pouch as it is sometimes called), is attached by adhesive to the stoma that collects the faeces. The opening on the abdominal wall must be cleaned regularly and the bag changed daily because the faeces can irritate the skin resulting in ulceration and infection. When a urostomy is performed, the bladder is replaced by a bag attached to a stoma to collect urine.

A Colostomy

The most common ostomy is a colostomy. If possible, the surgeon will simply remove the diseased part and join the two remaining healthy parts of the colon (large bowel) back together. If the damage is too extensive or if the damage is too near the end of the digestive tract, a colostomy is performed.

Most colostomies are *sigmoid colostomies*; the sigmoid colon is the part of the bowel that is passed through the abdominal wall and formed into a stoma. If necessary, a colostomy can be formed from any part of the large bowel. The faeces from a colostomy are usually firmer than that from an ileostomy. This is because the large bowel is still intact in colostomates and absorbs water passed through the stomach.

An Ileostomy

An Ileostomy is sometimes called a "Brooke's ileostomy" (after the British Surgeon, Bryan Brooke who devised the first ileostomy that really worked) or colectomy. It is a permanent opening from the small bowel, to allow

Unwanted Baggage

faeces to leave the body without passing through the large bowel. This operation usually involves the removal of the entire colon.

In some patients, the rectum and anus are also removed. If the rectum remains intact, patients may feel rectal spasms – the feeling of wanting to pass a motion. This is quite normal in the early days after the operation and may result in some discharge. The anus may continue to secrete a small amount of mucus that is harmlessly passed whenever the urge occurs.

The discharge into the bag is more liquid than faecal output from a colostomy. This is because there is no bowel to act as a distribution point for liquid intake. It is therefore vital that an ileostomate maintains a high level of hydration.

Dehydration is a serious problem for ileostomists. It occurs when the water content of your body is reduced leading to changes in the balance of chemical substances in the body, especially a lack of sodium (salt) and potassium. In order to function properly, many of the body's cells depend on these substances maintained at the correct levels.

A Kock or Koch internal pouch

A Kock or Koch pouch is a form of continent ileostomy. This is made possible by having an internal pouch constructed from the small intestine that stores the waste products until the person is ready to irrigate (see chapter on irrigation). A one-way nipple valve sitting flush with the skin stops the faeces from coming out at all other times.

In this way, a person avoids having to wear a bag and usually just has a stomal cap, or even a waterproof covering, to protect the stoma. Nipple valve slippage is a unique complication of the Kock's Pouch, making it difficult to irrigate or stop the faeces coming out spontaneously. If this occurs, surgery is then needed to correct it or replace the internal pouch with a full urostomy.

A Urostomy or IlealConduit

An **Ileal Conduit** is the most common permanent type of **Urostomy.** If surgical removal of the bladder is called for, a segment of small bowel is utilised to transfer urine directly from the kidneys and urethras through a stoma on the skin and into an external collection bag. It is this piece of intestine that is used for the stoma, like an ileostomy stoma. The only difference is that urine, instead of faeces is expelled into the bag.

Unwanted Baggage

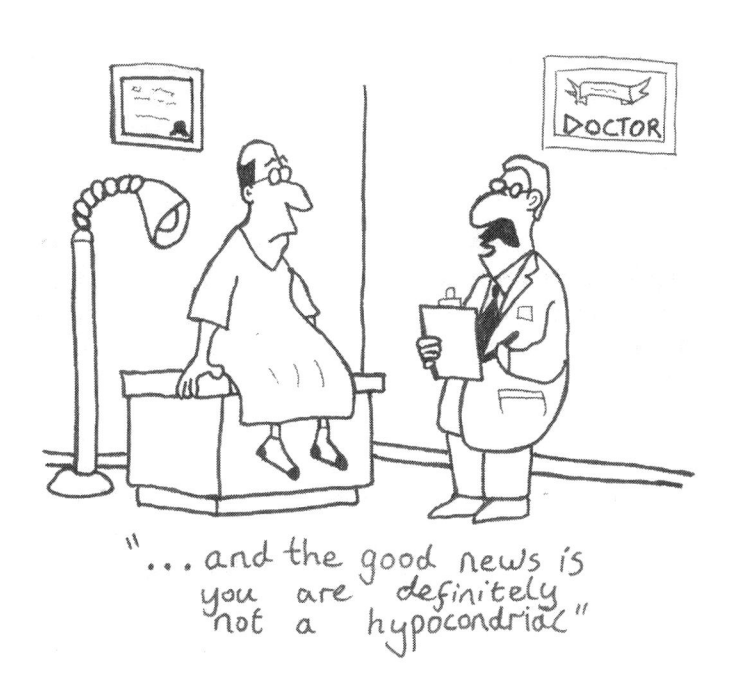

Chapter Three
Specific Symptoms and Treatments
...Finding a Diagnosis

I must make it clear that I am not a medical professional neither do I hold any medical qualifications. I am simply an ostomate with several years' patient experience.

The following information is a compilation of details found on a number of copyright free medical websites available to all.

If you are experiencing any of the problems listed, **it is imperative that you seek <u>professional medical advice</u>** as soon as possible.

Intimate problems are always embarrassing to discuss with anyone. However, early diagnosis is vital and can be life saving in the majority of cases of serious illnesses. Early treatment will prevent illness from becoming worse. A few moments of awkwardness with your doctor could put your mind at ease and on the road to treatment if it is necessary.

Crohn's Disease

Crohn's disease is a chronic, relapsing condition. Chronic means that it is ongoing. Relapsing means that there are

Unwanted Baggage

times when symptoms flare-up (relapse), and times when there are few or no symptoms (remission). The severity of symptoms, and how frequently they occur, varies from person to person.

Crohn's has become more common over the last twenty years. Although, it is not known whether this is due to new, efficient diagnosis, or if it is an indication that Crohn's is on the increase.

In Crohn's disease, patches of inflammation can develop in parts of the small intestine, large bowel and even the mouth, throat and stomach. A patch of inflammation may be small, or spread quite a distance along part of the gut. Several patches of inflammation may develop along the gut, with normal sections of gut in between. This patchy inflammation can impair diagnosis. Biopsies are taken, but the machinery may sometimes miss patches of inflammation through no fault of the operator. The patches may be just out of reach or on the opposite side to the fibre optic camera.

The exact causes of Crohn's are unknown. Although not strictly an inherited disease, about one in ten people with Crohn's disease have a close relative who also has it. This means there may be some genetic factor.

It is also know as an autoimmune disease. Our bodies have an immune system that protects us from disease and infection. However, if you have an autoimmune disease, your immune system attacks itself by mistake, and you will become seriously ill. Autoimmune diseases can affect connective tissue in your body (the tissue that binds together body tissues and organs). Autoimmune disease can affect many parts of your body, like your nerves, muscles, endocrine system (system that directs your body's hormones and other chemicals), and digestive system.

Other factors such as a virus may be involved. One theory is that a germ may trigger the immune system to cause inflammation in parts of the gut in people who are genetically prone to develop the disease.

As the disease emerges, the inflammation may cause one or more of the following:

- **Pain:** The site of the pain depends on which part of the gut is affected. The last part of the small intestine is the most usual site. Therefore, a common area of pain is the lower right side of the abdomen. When Crohn's disease first develops, it is sometimes mistaken for appendicitis. The severity of pain can vary from person to person. In addition, a sudden change or worsening of pain may indicate a complication.

- **Ulcers:** An ulcer is a raw area of the lining of the gut that may bleed. You may see blood when you pass faeces.

- **Diarrhoea:** This varies from mild to severe. The diarrhoea may contain pus or blood. An urgency to get to the toilet is common. A feeling of wanting to go to the toilet but with nothing to pass is also common.

- A feeling of being **generally unwell**, with a loss of appetite, weight loss, fever, and exhaustion.

- **Anaemia** may occur if you lose a lot of blood or fail to retain necessary nutrients.

- **Mouth ulcers** are common.

- **Anal fissures** may occur. These are painful 'cracks' in the skin of the anus. Skin tags (small fleshy wart-like lumps) may also appear around the anus.

With Crohn's disease, you may not have diarrhoea if the disease is just in the small intestine. A persistent pain in the abdomen, without any other symptoms may be due to a small patch of Crohn's disease in the small intestine. If large parts of the gut are affected, you may not absorb food well, and you may become deficient in vitamins and other nutrients.

In addition to the gut, other parts of the body are sometimes affected. These include inflammation, pain, and ulceration of some joints; skin rashes; red patches on the skin; inflammation of the eye (uveitis); and liver inflammation.

Oral Crohn's disease (orofacial granulomatosis) can manifest as occasional swollen and cracked lips, severe mouth ulcers and a rutted pattern inside the mouth. It does not however affect the teeth or gums and will not cause gum disease or teeth structure. A mouth X-ray will show jaw deformations that can be caused by Crohn's affect on the jawbones.

It is not clear why these problems occur. The immune system may trigger inflammation in other parts of the body when there is inflammation in the gut. These other problems tend to go when the gut symptoms settle, but not always.

Complications of Crohn's may occur, particularly if flare-ups are frequent or severe. These can include the following, which usually need treatment with surgery.

- **Stricture:** This is a narrowing of part of the gut. It is due to scar tissue that may form in the wall of an inflamed part of the gut. A stricture can cause difficulty in food passing through a blockage leading to pain and vomiting.

- **Perforation:** This small hole forms in the wall of the gut. The contents of the gut can then leak out and cause infection or an abscess inside the abdomen. This can be serious and life threatening.

- **Fistula:** This is when the inflammation causes a channel to form between two parts of the gut. For example, a fistula may form between parts of the small intestine with part of the colon. Fistulas can also form between part of the gut and other organs, such as the bladder or uterus. The contents of the gut may then leak into these other organs.

- **Cancer:** People with Crohn's disease have a small increased risk of developing cancer of the intestine (bowel cancer).

Unwanted Baggage

Depending on where the symptoms arise from, various tests can confirm the diagnosis, and determine how much of the gut is affected. A colonoscopy will allow biopsies to be taken from the lining of the gut.

A colonoscopy is a test to examine the colon. A colonoscope is a thin, flexible, telescope. It is passed through the anus and into the colon. It can be pushed all the way round the colon as far as the caecum (where the small and large intestine meet).

The colonoscope contains fibre optic channels that allows light to allow the operator to see inside your colon. The colonoscope also has a 'side channel', down which devices can be passed and which can then be manipulated by the operator. For example, the operator may take small samples (biopsies) from the inside lining of the colon by using a thin 'grabbing' instrument which is passed down the side channel. Air may also be passed into the colon to ease viewing.

If you have symptoms coming from the upper part of the gut, then a doctor may suggest an endoscopy.

An endoscopy is a test to examine the throat, stomach, and upper part of the gut. The endoscope operates in exactly the same way as the colonoscope, but passes through the mouth all the way into the gut. Again, biopsies can be taken through this.

For both colonoscopies and endoscopies, a light sedative or anaesthetic spray is usually offered. Most patients accept some sedation as the procedure can be quite uncomfortable and sometimes painful. There is no reason to suffer additional pain or discomfort, so ask the admitting staff or your consultant about this in advance. A special X-ray of the large intestine (barium enema), or small intestine (barium meal) may be advised. Barium coats the lining of the gut and shows up as white on X-ray films. Typical patterns on the films show which parts of the gut, if any, are affected. Either the patient can swallow the mixture or it can be administered through a naso-gastric tube with a mild anaesthetic.

CAT scans and standard MRI examinations are frequently used to support colonoscopy results. A Gel MRI can also be used to highlight areas of the small and large bowel to help pinpoint affected or problem areas. (These new MRI's are not available at all NHS hospitals).

Treatment for Crohn's disease is an evolving field. Various new medicines are under investigation and are likely to change the treatment strategies and options over the next few years. The NICE website details the latest medication and treatment available on the NHS.

www.nice.org.uk/search/guidancesearchresults.jsp?keywords=crohn%27s&searchType=guidance.

The most common treatment to control symptoms when Crohn's disease first develops is either a steroid or a 5-aminosalicylate medicine. Both of these types of medicine reduce inflammation, but work in different ways. Medication is prescribed for a few weeks until symptoms clear. A course of medication is then prescribed each time symptoms flare-up.

Unwanted Baggage

Treatment for flare-ups can include (but is not limited to):

- **A course of steroids** usually eases symptoms within four weeks of starting them. The dose is gradually reduced until symptoms ease.

- **5-aminosalicylate medicines** include sulfasalazine, mesalazine, ofsalazine, and balsalazide. They are an alternative to steroids, and often work well for mild or moderate flare-ups. They do not work in all cases.

- **Other 'second line' medicines**. These include certain antibiotics, biologics and immunosuppressive medicines. The success of these varies and a specialist may advise one or more to find the best medicine or combination of medicines.

- **Surgery** to remove a severely affected section or all of the gut may be needed if other treatments do not work. If all of the gut is removed, a stoma will be formed and an ostomy bag will then be necessary. Surgery is usually needed to treat complications such as fistulas, strictures, and abscesses.

Once an initial episode of symptoms has cleared, medication can be prescribed to prevent further episodes (flare-ups) of symptoms. For example, azathioprine or 6-mercaptopurine - some studies suggest that these may be better at preventing flare-ups than 5-aminosalicylate medicines. Methotrexate is another alternative that is sometimes used. This is administered initially by injection, usually on the chemotherapy ward and, if it proves to be successful in limiting flare-ups, then you or your carer can learn to administer this at home. Your doctor will advise about the pros and cons of these long-term medications.

A monthly blood test is essential to monitor iron, potassium and vitamin D and A.

There are certain general measures that can also help prevent flare-ups:

- If smokers are able to stop or cut down, it is believed that this may reduce the number of flare-ups.

- Control of liquid output: If this is left unchecked, it can irritate the gut. Anti-diarrhoeal medicines such as Imodium (or jelly babies / marshmallows / natural gelatine sweets) will help to thicken faecal output and can reduce liquid output.

- Follow a sensible low fibre diet. Eat little and often.

- Live as stress free a life as possible.

Some people believe that a 'trigger' may *possibly* cause symptoms to flare-up. Everyone is different, so what affects one patient may be harmless to another. Some patients have noted reactions to milk products, food preservatives, certain medicines such as aspirin or other anti-inflammatory medicines, or antibiotics. Stress is

Unwanted Baggage

also considered a major trigger that can cause flare-ups. However, it is difficult to prove whether such triggers are to blame, and in most cases, no change in diet or lifestyle is advised. A well-balanced, healthy diet is usually best. Little and often is the key to eating sensibly for any bowel or urinary disease.

There are no accurate statistics or comparative studies that show which patients are more prone to flare-ups. People with Crohn's disease may have frequent and/or severe flare-ups. A few people with Crohn's disease have just one or two flare-ups in their lifetime. The majority of people with Crohn's disease require surgery at some stage in their life for a complication. In about half of people with Crohn's disease, surgery is needed within the first 10 years of developing the disease. The most common reason for surgery is to relieve a stricture that has formed.

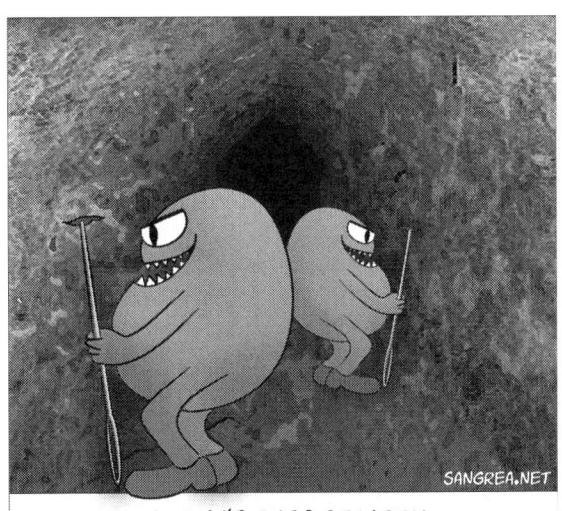

CROHN'S BUGS AT WORK

Ulcerative colitis (UC)

UC is a chronic, relapsing condition. Chronic means that it is persistent and ongoing. Relapsing means that there are times when symptoms flare-up, and times when there are few or no symptoms. The severity of symptoms, and how frequently they occur, varies from person to person. The first episode of symptoms is often the worst.

- **Colitis** means 'inflammation of the colon'.
- **Ulcerative** means that ulcers tend to develop. An ulcer is a raw area on the lining of the intestine that may bleed.

The causes of UC unknown. UC can affect anyone. About one in five people with UC have a close relative who also has UC, so, there may be some genetic factor. However, other factors such as a virus may trigger UC to develop. One theory is that a germ triggers the immune system to cause inflammation in the large intestine in people who are genetically prone to develop the disease.

About one person in a thousand in the UK develops UC. It can develop at any age but most commonly first emerges between the ages of fifteen and forty. About one in seven cases first develop in people over sixty.

In most cases, UC starts in the rectum. This causes a proctitis, which means 'inflammation of the rectum'. In some cases, it only affects the rectum, and the colon is not affected. In others, the disease spreads up to affect some or the entire colon. Between flare-ups, the inflamed areas of colon and rectum heal and symptoms go away. About half of people with UC have mild and infrequent

Unwanted Baggage

symptoms. The other half has more frequent flare-ups, with moderate or severe symptoms. During a flare-up, some people develop symptoms gradually. In others, the symptoms develop quite quickly. Symptoms are:

- **Diarrhoea:** This varies from mild to severe. The diarrhoea may contain mucus, blood or pus. An urgency to get to the toilet is common. A feeling of wanting to go to the toilet but with nothing to pass is also common (known as tenesmus). Water is not absorbed as well as it should be in the inflamed colon, which makes the diarrhoea watery.

- **Blood** mixed with diarrhoea is common ('bloody diarrhoea').

- **Cramp-like pains, primarily** in the abdominal area.

- **Pain,** when passing faeces.

- **Proctitis,** symptoms may be different if a flare-up only affects the rectum, and not the colon. You may have fresh bleeding from the rectum, and you may form normal faeces rather than have diarrhoea. You may even become constipated, but with a frequent feeling of wanting to go to the toilet.

- **A Feeling of being generally unwell** is typical if the flare-up affects a large amount of the large intestine, or lasts a long time. Fever, tiredness, feeling sick, weight loss, and anaemia may develop.

- **Other problems in addition to problems in the intestine and bowel can** occur in about one in ten cases. These can include skin rashes, inflammation of the eye (uveitis), pain and inflammation of some joints and liver inflammation. It is not clear why these occur. The immune system may trigger inflammation in other parts of the body when there is inflammation in the gut. These other problems tend to go when the abdominal symptoms settle, but not always.

- **A severe flare-up** is uncommon, but if it occurs, it can cause serious illness. The whole colon may become ulcerated, inflamed, and dilated. A part of the colon may perforate, or severe bleeding may occur. Surgery is often needed if a flare-up becomes severe (see below).

- **Cancer:** The risk of developing cancer of the colon may increase slightly if you have UC.

A colonoscopy will show the appearance of the inside lining of the colon. A small sample (biopsy) of the colon will be examined for the atypical pattern of the cells to confirm the diagnosis.

The common treatment to control symptoms when UC first develops is either a steroid or a 5-aminosalicylate medicine. Both of these types of medicine reduce inflammation, but work in different ways. While these are usually prescribed in tablet form, they can also be taken as an enema, if only the rectum and last part of the colon is affected. A course of medication is prescribed each time symptoms flare-up. Treatment for flare-ups can include (but is not limited to):

- **A course of steroids (corticosteroids)** will usually ease symptoms. The initial high dosage is gradually reduced. Once a flare-up is settled, steroids are not continued. This is because side effects may develop if steroids are prescribed for a long time (several months or more). The aim is to treat any flare-ups, but to keep the total amount of steroid treatment, over the years, as low as possible.

- **5-sminosalicylate medicines** include sulfasalazine, mesalazine, ofsalazine, and balsalazide. They are an alternative to steroids, and often work well for mild or moderate flare-ups. They do not work in all cases. Some people may need to switch to steroid medication if a 5-aminosalicylate medicine is not working, or if the flare-up is severe.

- **Other medicines** that suppress the immune system (immunosuppressants) can also be prescribed. If symptoms persist despite the above treatments., e.g. azathioprine or cyclosporine.

Once an initial episode of symptoms has cleared, additional prescribed medication may prevent further episodes (flare-ups) of symptoms. If you have UC and **do not** take a regular preventive medicine, you have about a seven in ten chance of having at least one flare-up each year. This may be reduced to a three in ten chance, if you take a preventative medication.

5-aminosalicylate medicines are commonly used to prevent flare-ups. A lower 'maintenance dose' than the dose used to treat a flare-up is usual. You can take one indefinitely to help keep symptoms at bay. Most people have little trouble taking these medicines. Some people develop side-affects such as abdominal pains, feeling sick, headaches, or rashes. If one medicine causes side-affects, switching to an alternative may be fine, as side effects can differ between the different 5-aminosalicylate medicines.

If a flare-up develops whilst you are taking a 5-aminosalicylate medicine then the symptoms will usually, quickly, ease if the dose is increased, or if you switch to a short course of steroids.

Other medicines may be advised if a 5-aminosalicylate medicine does not work. For example, either azathioprine or 6-mercaptopurine is sometimes used. About three in ten people with UC need surgery at some stage.

Surgery is considered in the following situations:

- **During a life-threatening flare-up**: Removing the large intestine may be the only option if it swells greatly, perforates, or bleeds uncontrollably.

- **If UC is not controlled by medication:** Some people remain in poor health with frequent flare-ups that do not settle properly. To remove the large intestine is a serious step, but for some people the operation is a relief after a long period of ill health.

Relationship between Ulcerative Colitis and Cancer of the Colon

The chance of developing cancer of the large intestine (colon) is slightly higher than average in people who have had UC for several years or more.

Because of this risk, people with UC are advised to have their large intestine routinely checked by means of regular colonoscopies.

Changes are usually seen in the biopsies, taken during the colonoscopies, long before any cancer develops. If changes are found, surgery to remove the large intestine is advised to prevent the cancer progressing.

Recent studies indicate that the risk of cancer is likely to be reduced in people who take regular long-term 5-aminosalicylate medication (described above).

Colorectal cancer

Colorectal cancer is a cancer of the colon or rectum. (It is sometimes called "Bowel Cancer" or "Cancer of the Large Intestine").

Despite the fact that this is one of the **most common cancers in the UK,** it does not attract the public attention that other cancers do probably because people avoid discussing nether regions! Additional publicity might serve to motivate the public into getting earlier checks for embarrassing problems. Colorectal cancer can affect any part of the colon or rectum, but most commonly first develops in the lower part of the descending colon, the sigmoid colon, or rectum. In most cases, colorectal cancer develops from a polyp formed on or within the lining of the colon or rectum.

A bowel polyp is a small growth that sometimes forms on the lining of the colon or rectum. Most bowel polyps develop in older people. About one in four people over the age of 50 develop at least one bowel polyp. Polyps are usually benign and cause no problems. However, sometimes a benign polyp can turn cancerous and most colorectal cancers develop from a polyp that has been present for five to fifteen years.

As the cancer cells multiply, they form a tumour. The tumour invades the wall of colon or rectum. Some cells may break off into the lymph channels or bloodstream. The cancer may then spread (metastasise) to lymph nodes nearby or to other areas of the body, most commonly the liver and lungs.

Although colorectal cancer can develop for no apparent reason, there are certain 'risk factors' that can increase the chance that colorectal cancer will develop. These include:

- **Ageing**: - Colorectal cancer is more common in older people. Most cases are in people over the age of 50.

- **Genetic** - If a close relative has had colorectal cancer

- If you have had **ulcerative colitis** (a condition of the colon) for more than 8-10 years.

- **Lifestyle factors** may be an additional contributory factor but there are no exact, proven tests. The NHS advises that any of the following may contribute to a vast number of illnesses: heavy smoking, excessive drinking and obesity.

When a colorectal cancer first develops and is small, it usually exhibits no symptoms. As it grows, the symptoms that develop can vary, depending on the site of the tumour. These symptoms are similar to those exhibited in most colon diseases. The most common symptoms to first develop are:

- **Bleeding.** You may see blood mixed with faeces (stools or motions). Sometimes the blood can make the faeces turn an unusually dark colour. The bleeding is not usually severe and not easily noticeable as it is just a small 'trickle', mixed with faeces. However, small amounts of bleeding that occur regularly can also lead to anaemia that can make you tired and pale.

- **Passing mucus** with faeces.

- **A dramatic change** from your usual 'bowel habit'. This means you may pass faeces more or less often than usual.

- **Diarrhoea or constipation** on a regular basis.
- A continual feeling of not **emptying the rectum** after passing faeces.
- **Abdominal pains**. These can be anything from mild to severe.

As the tumour grows in the colon or rectum, symptoms may increase. If the cancer spreads to other parts of the body, various other symptoms can develop. However, all the above symptoms may be due to a variety of other conditions, so tests are needed to confirm colorectal cancer.

If a doctor suspects that you may have colorectal cancer, he or she will examine you to look for signs such as a lump in your abdomen, anaemia, etc. The examination will usually include a rectal examination. However, often the examination is normal, especially if the cancer is in its early stages. Therefore, one or more of the following tests can be done:

- **A faecal occult blood test (FOB test).** A small sample of faeces is smeared onto a piece of card. A simple test can detect small amounts of blood in your faeces that you would not normally see with the naked eye. Occult means 'unseen' or 'invisible'. The FOB test can only say that you are bleeding from *somewhere* in the gut. It cannot tell from which part. Nor can it tell what is causing the bleeding. It is however, a useful test to confirm 'bleeding' within the gut.

Unwanted Baggage

- **Colonoscopy or flexible sigmoidoscopy.** This is similar to colonoscopy. The difference is that a shorter telescopic probe is used which is gently pushed into the rectum and sigmoid colon.

- **A biopsy** to remove a small sample of tissue from a part of the body. The sample is examined under the microscope to look for abnormal cells.

If you have confirmed to have colorectal cancer, further tests can assess if it has spread. These can include a CT scan, an MRI scan, or an ultrasound scan. The aim of these is to find out:

- How much the tumour in the colon or rectum has grown, and whether it has grown partially or fully through the wall of the colon or rectum.

- Whether the cancer has spread to local lymph nodes.

- Whether the cancer has spread to other areas of the body (metastasised).

A common prognosis staging system for colorectal cancer is called the Duke's classification. This is:

- Duke A: the cancer is just in the inner lining of the colon or rectum.

- Duke B: the cancer has grown to the muscle layer in the wall of the colon or rectum.

- Duke C: the cancer has spread to at least one lymph node near to the colon or rectum.

- Duke D: the cancer has spread to other parts of the body ('metastases' or secondary tumours). The most common sites for colorectal cancer to spread to are the liver and lungs.

If a polyp is found during a colonoscopy, it can often be easily removed. A removal utilises special fine instruments passed down side channels of the colonoscope. When the polyp is removed, it is microscopically examined. Most polyps do not contain cancer cells. However, removing the polyp prevents the risk that it may become cancerous sometime in the future. Some polyps do contain cancer cells. If these cells are confined within the polyp, the removal of the polyp is curative. If the cells have begun to spread to the wall of colon or rectum then an ostomy may be necessary to remove that section of colon or rectum.

Your specialist will advise on treatment options including surgery, chemotherapy and radiotherapy.

Without treatment, a colorectal cancer is likely get larger, and spread to other parts of the body. However, in many cases it grows slowly and may remain confined to the lining of the colon or rectum for some months before growing through the wall of the colon or rectum, or spreading.

If the cancer is diagnosed and treated at an early stage, there is a good chance of remission.

Unwanted Baggage

The treatment of cancer is a developing area of medicine. New treatments continue to be developed and the information on outlook above is very general.

The specialist who knows your case can give more accurate information about your particular outlook, and how well your type and stage of cancer is likely to respond to treatment.

Diverticular disease

Diverticular disease is an inflammation of the small sacs in the colon that can cause abscesses, scarring or perforation of the colon with peritonitis in severe cases.

A diverticulum is a small pouch with a narrow neck that protrudes (sticks out from) from the wall of the abdomen. Diverticula are more than one diverticulum. They can develop on any part of the intestinal system but usually occur in the colon. They most commonly develop in the section of the colon leading towards the rectum, where the stools are becoming more solid.

Diverticula are actually very common. They become more common with increasing age. About one in twenty people in their forties, about one in three people in their sixties, and about half of people in their eighties have Diverticular of the colon. Men and women are equally affected. The reason why Diverticula develop is not clear.

In most cases, Diverticula cause no harm or symptoms. If there is a problem symptoms will indicate this. They are as follows:

- **Pain** in the abdomen and/or bloating may occur. The pain is usually cramp-like and tends to come and go. You may get ease from pain and bloating by going to the toilet to pass stools.

- Constant **Diarrhoea or Constipation**.

If you have these symptoms with Diverticular, it is called 'Diverticular disease'.

Symptoms of Diverticular disease are similar to those that occur with a different condition called irritable bowel syndrome (IBS). However, IBS usually affects younger adults initially and so symptoms that first develop in a younger adult are more likely to be due to IBS. Likewise, symptoms that first develop in older people are more likely to be due to Diverticular disease. However, in some cases it is difficult to tell if symptoms are due to Diverticular disease or to IBS.

Complications are uncommon, and include the following. About one in ten people with Diverticula develop a bout of diverticulitis at some stage. This is when one or more of the Diverticula become inflamed and infected, which may occur if faeces become trapped and then stagnate in a Diverticula. Bacteria in the trapped faeces may then multiply and cause infection. Symptoms of diverticulitis include:

- A **constant pain** in the abdomen: It is commonly in the lower left side of the abdomen. This is over the site where Diverticular most commonly develop.

Unwanted Baggage

- **Fever** (high temperature).
- Continual Constipation **or diarrhoea**.
- You may have some **blood** mixed with your stools.
- You may experience **nausea** to varying degrees.

Antibiotics are commonly used to treat Diverticulitis and it usually responds well within a short time. If it the medication does not work, hospital admission is necessary, as surgery may be needed to drain an abscess or remove a badly infected part of the colon. Some people have several bouts of diverticulitis in their life.

Infected Diverticula occasionally cause a blockage of the colon, or forms a channel or fistula to other organs such as the bladder. Very rarely, a diverticulum may burst and cause infection inside the abdomen (peritonitis). Surgery is then needed to treat these complications.

Urostomies

Urostomy or urinary diversion is a surgically created opening in the abdomen that allows urine to pass directly out of the body. They are most commonly performed to remove bladder cancer, however, a urostomy may also be necessary where interstitial cystitis or some types of kidney disease are present, or if there is severe injury to the urinary tract. Urostomies generally have very little or no odour. Urine will collect throughout the day and night through an abdominal stoma.

Urostomies are usually performed because of:

- **Cancer:** – A cancerous growth in the bladder causing the removal or bypass of the entire bladder. The urine is then detoured through an abdominal stoma.

- **Congenital defects** that cause urine to back up into the kidneys, resulting in chronic infections.

- **Surgical Complications** because of non-related pelvic or abdominal surgery.

- Accidental **damage** to the bladder.

- Continual leakage from the bladder – **incontinence.**

Cancer of the bladder

About ten thousand people develop bladder cancer in the UK each year. In most cases, bladder cancer develops from the transitional cells that line the inside of the bladder. This type of cancer is called 'transitional cell bladder cancer'. Other types of bladder cancer are rare in the UK.

Transitional cell bladder cancer is divided into two groups:

- **Superficial tumours:** These occur in about four of every five cases. These tumours are confined to the inner lining, or just below the inside lining, of the bladder. Sometimes the

Unwanted Baggage

cells which form this type of cancer multiply to form little growths which stick out like 'warts' from the inside lining of the bladder.

- **Muscle invasive tumours.** These occur in about one in every five cases. These tumours have spread to the muscle layer of the bladder, or right through the wall of the bladder.

In many cases, the reason why a bladder cancer develops is unknown. However, there are factors that are known to increase the risk of bladder cancer developing. These include:

- **Increasing age**: Most bladder cancers occur in people over the age of fifty.

- **Smoking**: Bladder cancer is four times more common in smokers than in non-smokers. Chemicals from tobacco enter the body through inhalation, and these are expelled in urine. These specific chemicals in the urine are carcinogenic and highly damaging to the bladder cells. It is estimated that about one third of all bladder cancers are related to smoking.

- **Other chemicals:** Recent research has shown that certain workplace and environmental chemicals have also been linked to bladder cancer. Fortunately, many of these identified chemicals are now banned in the UK. However, bladder cancer may develop as late as ten to twenty years after exposure. Cases are still being diagnosed in people who worked with these chemicals many years ago.

- **Gender**: Bladder cancer is about three times as common in men as in women.

- **Schistosomiasis:** This is a bladder infection caused by a parasite that infests some Asian, African and South American countries.

- Repeated bouts of other types of **bladder infection** may also slightly increase the risk.

Symptoms of bladder cancer can include:

- **Blood in urine** or haematuria caused by an early bladder tumour. This is not usually painful. The blood in the urine may 'come and go' as the tumour bleeds from time to time.

- Frequent **passing of urine** or **pain** on passing urine: These symptoms are also quite common indicators of ordinary urine infections such as cystitis. If you experience this problem, always take a sample to your GP who will test it on the spot to confirm diagnosis.

- If the cancer is a muscle invasive type, and grows through the wall of the bladder, then other symptoms may develop over time. For example, pain in the lower abdomen.

Diagnosis is confirmed by:

- *Urine microscopy:* A sample of urine can examined for cancerous cells under the microscope. This test may detect cancer cells. However, if no cancer cells are found, it does not necessarily rule out bladder cancer. Further tests are often needed to confirm or rule out the diagnosis if symptoms continue.

- *Cystoscopy:* This test can confirm a bladder tumour. A cystoscopy allows a bladder specialist (urologist) to look into the bladder with a special thin telescope called a cystoscope. The cystoscope is eased into the bladder via the urethra. A cystoscopy is performed to look into the bladder and is normally done under local anaesthetic. If any additional procedure is done via the cystoscope, such as removing a tumour, then a general anaesthetic is used. An ultrasound may also be used to get an overall picture of the bladder.

During cystoscopy, an urologist can:

- See any areas on the lining of the bladder that look abnormal.

- Take biopsies of suspicious areas. The sample is then examined under the microscope to look for abnormal cells.

- Remove a superficial tumour with instruments that can be passed down a side channel of the cystoscope.

If you have a muscle invasive tumour, then further tests will assess if the cancer has spread. This assessment is 'staging' of the cancer. The aim of staging is to find out:

- How much the tumour in the bladder has grown, and whether it has grown to the edge, or through the outer part of the bladder wall.

- Whether the cancer has spread to local lymph nodes.

- Whether the cancer has spread to other areas of the body (metastasised).

Treatment

An operation to remove the bladder is the most common treatment. This is a major operation. You will need an alternative way of passing urine if you have your bladder removed this is by a 'urostomy'. A stoma will be formed to collect urine externally. An alternative operation may also be possible where the surgeon creates an artificial type of bladder from a part of the gut.

Incontinence

Urinary incontinence is the unintentional passing of urine. This very common problem affects about three million people in the UK.

In cases of **severe incontinence**, a urostomy may be performed to give the patient relief from continuous wetting and the skin problems associated with it.

Anyone can experience urinary incontinence. The condition affects far more women than men, and it occurs, to differing degrees, in one in five women who are over forty.

It may also be a temporary condition, for example when sneezing, stretching or involuntary or unexpected movement. Pelvic floor exercises may sometimes help this temporary condition.

There are various types of urinary incontinence, but the two main types are **stress incontinence** and **urge incontinence:**

Stress incontinence

This occurs when the pelvic floor muscles are too weak to prevent urination. The causes of this are:

When your pelvic floor muscles have been weakened, and you can no longer keep your urethra fully closed. Any sudden extra pressure on your bladder, such as laughing, sneezing, or orgasm can cause urine to leak out of your urethra.

A number of different factors can weaken your pelvic floor muscles.

Pregnancy and childbirth - this can sometimes overstretch, and strain, your muscles. It can cause a temporary or permanent condition

- **Menopause** - a lack of the hormone, oestrogen, can weaken your muscles

- **A hysterectomy (removal of the womb)** - this type of surgery can sometimes damage your muscles.

- **Age** - as you get older, your muscles naturally become weaker.

- **Obesity** - being obese can put excess stress on your muscles.

Urge incontinence

This occurs because of incorrect signals sent between the brain and the bladder. If you have urge incontinence, you may feel a sudden, intense need to pass urine, before releasing large amounts of urine. There is often only a few seconds between the need to urinate and the release of urine.

Your need to pass urine may be triggered by a sudden change of position, or even by the sound of running water. You may also find that you pass urine during sex, particularly when you reach orgasm.

If it is not possible to find a cause for urge incontinence, the problem may be diagnosed as 'overactive bladder syndrome'. However, some specific causes of urge incontinence have been identified:

- **Chronic Urine infections** - such as persistent cystitis (inflammation of the bladder lining).

Unwanted Baggage

- **Conditions that affect the nervous system** such as Parkinson's disease, multiple sclerosis, and stroke.

- **An enlarged prostate gland in men** - this can irritate your urethra (urinary opening) and lower bladder

These two types of urinary incontinence are responsible for up to 90% of all cases of the condition. It is also possible to have a mixture of both stress and urge urinary incontinence. The other 10% of cases are:

Overflow incontinence

This involves small trickles of urine when the bladder is full. Emptying the bladder more frequently can improve this condition. It may also feel as though your bladder is never fully empty, and you cannot empty it even when you try. This occurs when the muscles around the bladder are not able to squeeze the bladder empty. Causes of overflow incontinence:

- Nerve or muscle damage, perhaps caused by injury, or incidental result of surgery.

- Disease - such as Parkinson's disease, Multiple Sclerosis and Spina Bifida.

- An obstruction that makes it more difficult for your bladder to squeeze out all the urine that it contains. This obstruction can be caused by an enlarged prostate in men or by constipation or stricture of the urethra in either men or women.

As you are not able to empty the urine completely, your bladder and its muscles can become slack and are less able to be controlled. With larger amounts of urine retained in the bladder there is a chance that some urine will leak out when you do not want it to

Total incontinence

This is where there is no control of the urine flow and it is may be continuous. It can occur because of a congenital bladder disorder, or after surgery, or following an injury to the bladder area. Total incontinence may cause you to constantly pass large amounts of urine, even at night. You may also pass large amounts of urine every so often and leak small amounts in between.

This condition can be caused by

A bladder defect that you were born with.

- **An Injury to the spinal cord** which can disrupt the nerve signals between the brain and the bladder.
- **A bladder fistula** which is a small, tunnel-like structure, that can develop between the bladder, and/or a nearby area, such as the vagina.

Urinary incontinence of any kind can be an uncomfortable and upsetting problem. Many people may think that it is an inevitable part of aging, but there are several forms of treatment, including therapy, exercises, medicines and

Unwanted Baggage

electrical stimulation. Simple surgical procedures may also be successful in correcting age-related incontinence.

Ultimately, a urostomy is performed if all else fails. Patients who have experienced years of embarrassment, skin disorders, waterproof bedding and continuous changes of clothing, pads etc. will find a urostomy a welcome relief. A stoma is formed on the abdominal wall and urine then collects in a bag that can be emptied when full.

Chapter Four
If Surgery Is Necessary
...From Hospital Admittance to Discharge

Once surgery is scheduled, you should request a pre-operative visit with a "stoma nurse" - more correctly referred to as a specialist, colorectal nurse.

The nurse will spend some time with you either at hospital or at home. During this initial visit, tests will be conducted on skin sensitivity. This is a simple case of sticking small samples of a variety of bag adhesives onto your skin. They are left for a few days, then removed and any red rashes or skin sensitivities to certain brands will be noted. Most bag adhesives are very hypoallergenic and sensitivity is rare. However, if you are allergic to certain brands there are Barrier Skin Creams, Wipes and Sprays that form a seal to prevent the adhesive from touching the skin and do not compromise bag security.

During your initial visit, you will see your first few bags. You will be shown different styles - drainable or closed, one-piece or two-piece, large or small bags etc. You are not making a permanent choice of bag. Your stoma will change in shape and depth during your life and new products come onto the market all the time. Keep your options continually open.

Unwanted Baggage

You will be anxious about the whole procedure, and the idea of an ostomy itself, but the most important part of this early meeting will be to establish the location of the Stoma. You need to consider the clothes you wear. The last thing you need is a tight waistband constantly rubbing against the stoma.

The Stoma Nurse may ask you to lie down, sit down and crouch, to try to find the best possible position for your Stoma. If you disagree with the positioning, say so, as that will not be the only place it can go. You must avoid areas around old scars, natural creases, and your navel. It is best to make a good compromise between your personal preference and expert advice. It is crucial that the Stoma is easily accessible. After the operation, you will need to be able to see and reach the Stoma clearly to clean the area and change your bag.

If however, you are admitted for emergency ostomy surgery, the hospital stoma nurse may have time to run through these things with you prior to the operation. If not, the surgeon will make the best possible choice of stoma location.

Your life will be changing because of this operation so it is essential to plan as much as you can to help yourself through this difficult learning curve.

Remember that, in cases of permanent ostomies, you will be out of commission for some time. Organize your life! Schedule appointments and take care of business as much as possible in the weeks prior to surgery.

Approaching surgery with a positive attitude is important. To gain a good perspective talk to other people who have had the same procedure done. Your stoma nurse or the Colostomy, Ileostomy, Urostomy Associations can put you in touch with other stoma patients in your area. Other people's success stories can ease your mind and help you understand what is to come:

The Colostomy Association
www.colostomyassociation.org.uk

The Ileostomy Association
www.the-ia.org.uk

The Urostomy Association
www.uagbi.org.uk

Before you have the operation, you should recognise that pain and your general health deterioration have diminished your quality of life. Think and plan to life beyond surgery. It is very normal to feel increasingly tense and anxious as the surgery date approaches, so keep your mind busy and actively prepare for your hospital stay.

Pack your hospital case with care and estimate a 10-21 day stay. Your will need:

- Enough **pyjamas/nightwear** to change every day. There are always hospital gowns for emergencies - bags may burst or leak so extra clothing should be on hand at all times. A **dressing gown** can also hide a lot! Your partner/carer/family or friends may be able

Unwanted Baggage

to help launder nightwear between changes to reduce the amount you need to take in with you.

- You will not be able to wear your usual underwear. The hospital may provide **disposable underpants** – do ask them in advance. These are also useful in the three months following surgery as your stoma adjusts in size and shape. One of the cheapest suppliers on the internet is at: **www.justgloves.co.uk**

- You can also pre-order stoma **cotton underwear.** A limited selection is available on prescription -(maximum: six pairs/year.) Contact the suppliers for details and they will arrange for a prescription to be signed by your GP. You can also purchase them from the ostomy clothing manufacturers. See the suppliers in Chapter 14 for a full listing). However, do order one size larger than you would normally buy, as they will have to accommodate the new bag.

- **Toiletries etc**: The hospital will provide bags and stoma essentials. Although the bag adequately contains any odour, you may feel better having some scented products on hand.

- **Entertainment:** Although you may not feel like doing anything but sleeping for a few days, you will soon find that music, books, magazines, audio CDs or an Ipod will help distract your mind!

- **Writing materials:** You may want to write letters, do crosswords, other puzzles or keep notes on medication, physiotherapy etc.

- Keep a small amount of **cash** for phone calls /newspapers etc. Some hospitals now allow mobile phones that are much cheaper than using the hospital coin telephones. (You may wish to check on this beforehand.) All hospitals ask that you not bring credit/debit cards into hospital and that the amount of cash you keep on hand is minimal. Unfortunately, tests, operations and even visits to the bathroom mean that you are away from your locker. Most of these lockers are standard hospital issue and the only lockable compartment is reserved for medications.

- **Slippers:** As the floors are frequently washed and may be wet or slippery, you will need these to get to and from the bathroom and toilet.

Remember the hospital is not responsible for your property and you will be asked to sign a form acknowledging this. Do not take expensive items with you. All jewellery, glasses, contact lenses and dentures must be removed during surgery (apart from wedding bands).

Cultural Diversity

There are certain important restrictions that can affect patients undergoing surgery. Medical Staff should be made aware of these restrictions and act accordingly as much as they are able. The following are some simple guidelines – faith Ministers will advise when necessary.

Most hospitals provide chapels, prayer rooms or quiet rooms for visitors. Hospital Chaplains have access to Ministers of all faiths as appropriate, and they will attend a patient upon request. Patients' own faith advisors and Minsters are welcome to attend patients in hospital. Some religions ask that discretion be used when it comes to examining female patients.

Cleanliness is important to most religions but some have important cleanliness rituals in preparation for surgery, after surgery, before, after meals, and at prayer times. It is important that access to washing facilities be made available to these patients at these times.

Islamic Patients
Under Islam during Ramadan, no medication, food or drink is usually permitted but rules may be relaxed for seriously ill patients. However, at Prayer times, it is essential that a stoma bag be empty in keeping with the cleanliness ritual.

Hinduism
Hindus may not remove Sacred Threads or items on black cord as these are worn for protection during and after surgery. Tomatoes and citrus fruits are regarded as a hindrance to healing.

Judaism
Jewish patients will be offered their own dietary menus in most hospitals. Orthodox Jewish patients will normally attend faith hospitals. If none is available, then their rabbi will advise on diet and Shabbat rituals. Orthodox Jewish Women may wish to retain head covering, even when unconscious.

Sikhism
Many Sikhs are vegetarian and may accept a hospital vegetarian menu. However, many will prefer food to be brought from home including china and silverware. Medication that contains animal gelatine may be refused. Other forms of medication containing vegetarian gelatine are available.

Prayer & the Stoma
In terms of prayer, the surgeon/stoma nurse should be advised on prayer methods in order to ensure that the positioning of the stoma does not interfere with the ability to assume the correct prayer position.

Refusal of Surgical Procedures.
Jehovah's Witnesses and some other religions may forbid or at the least frown on surgical procedures. While very effort will be made on the patient's behalf to avoid surgery, it may become a last resort. Should a patient refuse surgery, there is little a medical professional can do, unless the patient is a minor or recognised as mentally incapacitated. Judicial remedies are open to surgeons treating minors in cases where parents refuse surgery.

Admission, surgery and recovery

Once admitted, you will be fitted with hospital wristbands and your ward staff will introduce themselves and begin the endless round of blood pressure, pulse and temperature readings that will become a regular part of your stay. An IV line will be inserted for all matter of necessary fluids.

If your operation is imminent, you will be on a nil-by-mouth regime. If you are allowed to eat, then try to manage as much as you are able, because you will need all your strength in the days to come.

Your stoma nurse will visit you to discuss your expectations and more importantly draw in indelible maker, the selected site of your stoma.

The surgeon will visit to brief you on the intricacies of the operation and on what to expect when you wake up from surgery. This will be the last time you will see him before the operation and it is the best time to iron out any final worries or ask any last questions you may have about the procedure.

The anaesthetist may also pay you a visit. Most of the information they need about anaesthetic allergies etc. have already been noted. However, some anaesthetists like to introduce themselves to the patient on the ward before they are taken to theatre.

When the theatre is ready, you will be wheeled on your bed down to pre-op. You will not be taken straight into the theatre, but to an adjacent room where the Anaesthetist will hook you up to a whole array of equipment to monitor your functions throughout surgery and for a short time afterwards. Your nametag will be checked and you will be asked to confirm your name, address and date-of-birth.

A syringe full of anaesthetic will be injected into your arm via the cannula (your IV line). You will soon drift off into to a deep sleep for the duration of the operation that will usually last four to five hours.

You will wake up in the recovery room. The surgery team will ask you if you are in any pain and if so, where you feel it most. If you are in pain, you will be given medication. You will not be moved from the recovery room until you are 'stable'. In other words: in no pain, fully awake and conscious of your surroundings. You will then be taken to a high dependency unit, where highly trained staff will constantly monitor your general condition for a few days. This is perfectly normal after major surgery. You may be aware of tubes from your neck, nose, arms and wound site. You will have a urinary catheter as you will be unable to move for while - this is all normal. Everything will all be disconnected as soon as reasonably possible.

Your family may be allowed to visit at unrestricted times, but only for short periods. You may not be fully conscious of your surroundings or events for up to forty-eight hours. The ward nurses will come to have a look at your stoma regularly to check everything is normal. You may be very anxious about the stoma but you may feel better waiting a few days before examining the stoma yourself.

You will be given intravenous post-operative antibiotics to ensure sure that no infection forms in any of the wound

Unwanted Baggage

areas. Try to sleep as much as possible; rest is always the best healer.

When you do come around properly, you will be aware of the number of the tubes leading from your body. This is quite a frightening moment until you realise the reason for their positioning.

- There will be a Saline drip tube attached to your arm to prevent dehydration, as you may not be allowed to eat for a few days.

- There will also be a drain leading from the wound itself, with a small bottle on the end to catch any blood or matter.

- A very fine tube up your nose and down into the stomach, preventing you from vomiting. You may also have tubes leading from the neck to administer medication. An oxygen mask may also be on hand.

- Finally, there may be a catheter fitted to drain the urine from your bladder (not in urostomies), as it is important for the nursing staff to monitor your output and it will prevent disturbing you to use a bedpan.

The daily ward routine will carry on around you while you rest. The surgical team will call on their rounds to see how your recovery is progressing. The ward nurses will take your blood pressure, pulse and temperature frequently. The nurse will have a look at the Stoma and check your wound sites. Your abdomen will be quite bruised and the wound sites may be heavily bandaged. The nurses will not remove any appliances for the first day to give everything a chance to settle down.

Over the next few days, you will gradually return to the real world. You will graduate from bed baths to visiting the bathroom, from lying to sitting, from sitting in a chair to beginning to walk around.

You will watch as the nurses change the ostomy bags and later, under guidance from the stoma nurse you can try this yourself. However, you will probably feel very weary for the next couple of weeks, and it is important to let nature take its course and not to rush into anything.

Ask for painkillers, as you need them. There is no need to suffer any undue pain. Initially you will be given painkillers regularly and you will be attached to a special machine via your IV. By pressing a button, you will be able to administer a single dose of morphine to control the pain as you feel the need. The machine administers an exact dose and it may only be used at pre-set intervals so there is no danger of an accidental overdose. The nursing staff will explain how to use this effectively and to ensure that you are pain free.

You should move as much as you are able to help your circulation. If for any reason you are still confined to bed, just move your limbs, wriggle your feet and bend your knees. The hospital will provide special socks and daily injections to prevent Deep Vein Thrombosis. The socks may feel uncomfortable at first – ask the nursing staff to pull the toes slightly so they are not too constrictive and this will prevent a feeling of itching.

Unwanted Baggage

Many ostomy patients will not have been eating properly for months so even hospital food will come as a pleasant surprise! It is very, very important to eat little and often.

A Physiotherapist will visit you to talk through any concerns you may have about mobility.

It is important not to view the recovery period as time wasted, but rather, as time to rest and recuperate. Time invested in the rehabilitation process is necessary for your recovery.

The stoma nurse will be a regular visitor towards the end of your hospital stay. She will be there to guide and help you with your bag and in cleaning the stoma. You will not be expected to do everything all at once.

If you wish, the hospital Chaplain will visit and pray with you. You have had traumatic surgery and the Chaplain is used to helping people cope through the early, frightening days of post-operative experience. They are on hand for patients and relatives or friends as the need arises so ask the nursing staff if you wish to see him/her.

The average length of stay after open bowel surgery is between ten and twenty-one days. As you can imagine it is very much up to your own healing speed. There are no set rules for this. Usually once your stitches are removed, you can go home, (although some may remain in place after you are discharged). The district nurse will call to your home and remove any that remain.

The average length of stay after Keyhole bowel surgery is around five to six days or so. Again, this could be more or less, depending on how you progress. (Keyhole surgery is usually only used for temporary colostomies while the bowel is resting).

During your stay, you will be surprised how quickly you recover. Visitors are encouraged and may help make time pass quickly. Each ward has its own phone number so that family and friends can check on your progress. A number of hospitals no longer allow flowers or plants so do not be disappointed if you do not receive any! Most wards are now specialised, comprised of people who have had similar surgeries so you can exchange experiences. It is good to talk to other people who know exactly how you are feeling.

Hospital Discharge

You will be discharged when a number of things are in place:

- You are not in pain, or you are happy that your pain can be controlled by medication.
- The stoma is working properly.
- You are eating and drinking reasonably well.

You will need someone to drive you home and be on hand at home to help you when you arrive. If this is not possible, hospital staff will arrange transport for you.

If you live alone, Social Services will meet with you while you are in hospital to arrange for care service to visit you on a regular basis to help with dressing and bathing and

Unwanted Baggage

they will organise meals-on-wheels until you are able to cope without support. In some instances, you may be transferred temporarily to a cottage hospital before eventually being discharged home.

When you are discharged, you will be given numerous items:

- **Your prescriptions**. - These will vary dependent upon individual patient needs. **Letters** for your doctor and the district nurses may be sent directly or handed to you to pass on.

- **A Post-operative surgical appointment**. - The ward nurse will make this for you, usually for four to six weeks after your discharge.

- The hospital will arrange for you to be visited by the District Nurse upon your arrival at home and for several days over the following two weeks dependent upon your personal needs. This is essential, as they will clean and dress the wound sites and help with the stoma .

- The hospital stoma nurse will also arrange for your local stoma nurse to visit on your first day home and regularly for a few weeks.

- The most important item given to you at discharge is your **discharge pack from the Stoma Nurse**. Inside will be enough appliances and supplies to last for two weeks after you leave hospital. Your local stoma nurse will then re-order for you and then instruct you into your preferred ordering process. You may also simply order items from the local chemist through a simple repeat prescription from your doctor, although a door-to-door, discreet delivery service is very handy and much easier to manage through on-line or telephone ordering.

- All ostomy supplies are free including bags, accessories, wipes, creams, lotions and sprays regardless of price or manufacturer of choice. Underwear and bag covers, girdles, stoma caps bed pads and waterproof mattress covers and belts are all prescription items.

- The most important leaflet is a **prescription exemption form**. In the UK, permanent Ostomists qualify for free prescriptions (temporary Ostomists qualify, whilst you have a Stoma). If you are resident in Wales or Scotland, under eighteen, in full time education or in receipt of benefits, you will qualify anyway but you will still need to complete the form to order supplies from England and Northern Ireland. You will need to complete this as soon as possible and hand it to your district nurse who will arrange for your GP to fill in the type of exemption. The practice will most probably send the form off for you. You will then receive a permanent prescription exemption certificate.

Unwanted Baggage

- Other leaflets for you may include details of the various medical associations and any local support groups.

- Finally, you will be given a supply of cleaning wipes and disposal bags for used appliances. These are complementary from an Ostomy Supplies Home Delivery Company and they will make sure their registration form is in the pack. There are many of these that offer differing degrees of efficiency and service. You are free to choose your own. (See Chapter 14: suppliers).

Never lose sight of your goals. The surgeon and surgical team have done their work in the operating room - the rest is up to you. Be inspired and work hard during the rehabilitation phase of your recovery.

Returning home

This is another new adventure. You will feel tired and will need to rest a lot. You **must not lift anything heavier than a full kettle for at least three months**. In the early stages (three – six months), you must be very careful to avoid stretching, lifting and bending or you may cause a parastomal hernia.

Even if you feel on top of the world, take life easy, begin things gradually and let friends and family wait upon you. Enjoy being pampered and spoilt and you will feel so much better. After all, you have undergone life-changing surgery and your body and mind will need time to adapt.

Chapter Five
The Stoma Nurse
...Meeting Your New Best Friend

The stoma and colorectal care service was established in the UK in the early 1970s by Barbara Saunders. It followed an example that was set up in the United States in 1953. By providing such a service, the NHS has recognised that there are special needs of people undergoing colorectal surgery resulting in a stoma, beyond that of standard nursing care.

Colorectal and Stoma nurses are highly trained, specialised professionals who provide acute and rehabilitative needs for people with selected disorders of the gastrointestinal and genitourinary systems. This means that they provide direct care to people with abdominal stomas, wounds, fistulas, drains, pressure ulcers, and/or continence disorders. They not only provide nursing care but also combine that with teaching and counselling on all stoma related topics.

There are currently several hundred qualified stoma and colorectal nurses in the UK. The stoma nurse is trained to assist patients in hospital pre and post surgery, and thereafter, to visit the new ostomate at home on a regular basis.

Unwanted Baggage

Your stoma nurse will give you advice on all aspects of stoma care such as bag changing, dietary advice, and advice on cleaning of the skin surrounding the attached collection bag, appliances and other supplies.

One of the most important ways in which the stoma nurse can support a patient is to teach a patient in such a way as to ensure their independence.

The stoma nurse will always be patient, empathetic and compassionate. At first, they will liaise with the district nurses as their focus is on your stoma maintenance whereas the district nurse will take responsibility for your wound care.

Beyond this educational role, the stoma nurse acts as a counsellor and will help the ostomate through the gamut of emotions that they are bound to feel. They are also able to offer advice on any intimate matters about which you must not be afraid to ask. If they feel they are unable to help in any way, or if they are concerned, they will refer you to your GP or arrange for additional psychological counselling.

They will not hesitate to refer you back to the hospital or your GP if they think there are serious problems with the stoma or believe you may be heading for a relapse.

After initial regular visits during your first few months, your stoma nurse will take a background role. She will leave her contact numbers and make sure you know that you can call her at any time if you are worried about anything physical or emotional. These incredible nurses devote and inordinate amount of time to all their patients and are never to busy to offer a few words of reassurance.

Elizabeth Prosser & Philip Prosser

They are an invaluable resource and one with which you will become comfortable.

Personally, I would like to thank my own colorectal nurse, Mary Platt, for her incredible patience as we tried out heaps of bags and adhesives. Her sense of humour really helped me to see things differently. She was always on the end of a phone when I needed her advice. Mary takes an active part not only in helping all her patients, but also in fundraising for the local branches of the colon cancer charity, the colorectal association and CROHN'S AND COLITIS UK. *(note: The illustration below is not Mary!!!)*

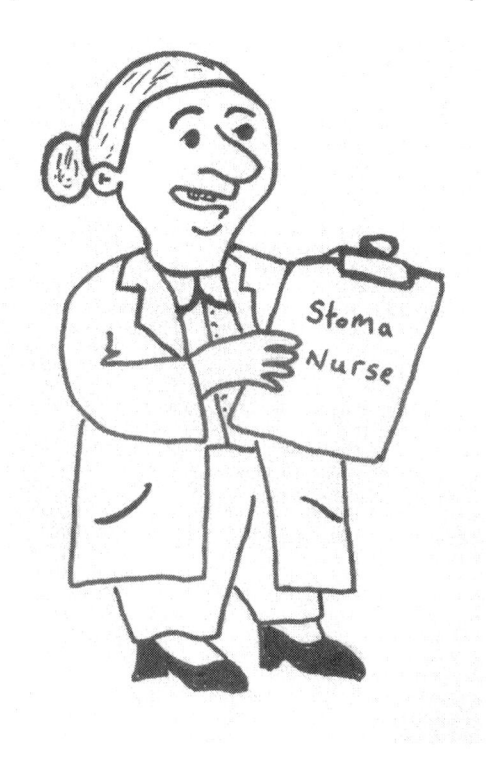

Chapter Six
Early Days
...The Beginning of Life after Surgery.

When you are discharged, it is essential that you listen to the district nurses who will be attending your wound care and to the stoma nurse who will be seeing to your stoma.

The other person you must listen to is you – or rather your body. You have had a major, serious operation. You must do only what your body will let you. If you are tired, simply lie down and go to sleep. Even closing your eyes will help. In sleep, there is recovery. As soon as you feel well enough, potter around, do a few things, but stop as soon as your body gives warning signals. Under no circumstances, lift anything heavier than a full kettle. Do not stretch or bend at all.

All stoma patients will experience initial physical problems. In the first instance do not hesitate do seek advice from your stoma nurse. Do not wait to get help, as your stoma is new and it will change quite dramatically in shape and size over the first few months. These changes affect the bag seal and if you do not change your bag accordingly, you will experience leaks and soreness.

You can order your pouches to be pre-cut by the manufacturer. Ask your stoma nurse to measure and cut a template for them to use. This system is much easier than trying to cut your own bag each time you need to change it.

Scars differ from person to person. Those who have had keyhole surgery are the lucky ones. The rest of us will have to do some work to ensure that the scars minimalise over the next couple of months. If you notice any slight swelling or discolouring in the scar area, point this out to your district or stoma nurse, as there may be a slight infection. If any scars feel uncomfortable, then **sudocrem™** is a wonderful antiseptic cream available at most high street chemists. Any generic Lavender oil can be used to massage into the scar area that should make the skin softer and heal quicker. Bio-oil™ is also recommended for tissue healing, well known to new mothers with stretch marks!

Establish a daily Routine

Life with a stoma is different. You should build a routine to attend to bag changing, cleaning, emptying the bag and adapting your life in general. A bag has not made you different; it is just an extra chore to take care of. Just as you routinely wash your face, apply make-up, wash your hair, shave – attending to the stoma will become just another step in your daily routine.

Initially, you can expect to be quite slow at changing your appliance. As with most things in life, the more you practice, the faster you will get. Single piece bags usually

Unwanted Baggage

need to be changed every twenty-four hours. Pick the best time in the day for you to do this - ideally, it should be at least four hours after a meal. Remember you will need "undisturbed toilet time" for the duration of the bag change

You do not necessarily have to change in the bathroom, you can use your bedroom if you are more comfortable - just have a small bowl of warm water ready before you begin. Most people seem to prefer the bathroom as it is a completely private place and has easy access to constant warm water and a toilet in case of emergency.

It is a good idea you to get a container in which you can keep all your supplies and a few pouches. An ice cream container is ideal. If you use a home delivery service for your supplies, they will send you a complementary selection of specially designed, lined bags for travel use.

Prepare everything before you even consider removing the appliance, as you can guarantee the stoma will "fountain" while you are at your most vulnerable! Lay everything you need out, open sachets etc. and put everything where you can easily reach It. If you warm the bag on a nearby radiator (adhesive side down), while you are washing the stoma, the adhesive sticks better.

I strongly recommend that you let the manufacturer pre-cut the bags to size, as, this will ensure that there will be no rough edges when they are machine cut. If you wish to cut your own shape, make a template first that fits snugly around the stoma. Use the template to cut the bags. Your Stoma Nurse will either make a template for you or show you how to do it.

Gentlemen may need to shave the area around the stoma to remove body hair from the abdomen. Be careful not to catch the stoma with the blade. Any longer hair on the stoma edge is better removed with rounded end scissors.

The optimum time for changing is four hours after any meal but the stoma is unpredictable. You can guarantee that it will leak as soon as you decide to change bags! See Chapter 14 for individual products.

- With your flange or pouch cut to size, you are now ready to remove your current appliance. You can sit on the closed toilet seat or small stool, lower your trousers/skirt and underwear to knee level (or remove completely) and protect with a towel. Using a laundry peg, pin up your top away from the stoma area.

- Place a dry wipe (supplied free from your bag suppliers) or good quality kitchen towel on the thigh under the bag. This will catch any sudden leaks or spills.

- Using an adhesive remover aerosol, carefully peel away the adhesive from the skin, working off any bits that may resist with a cotton swab or dry wipe. Do not use toilet tissue or cotton wool as this may flake off and enter the stoma opening.

After the bag has been removed, use an adhesive remover cloth (supplied in sachets), to remove any excess adhesive. Have a dry wipe on hand to cover the stoma

Unwanted Baggage

opening to mop up any excretions. Wet a dry wipe with warm water and clean the skin around the stoma . Soap is not necessary but you may wish to use it. Ensure you rinse off the remains of the adhesive remover. Do not use any cosmetic alcohol based skin cleanser/lotion. Dansac currently make the only approved skin lotion cleanser that can be used after washing; It is an excellent product. If you prefer you can use a wet wipe instead of water (provided free by the bag suppliers). Carefully wipe the stoma so it is completely clean. Try not to rub too hard, as the fragile stoma will begin to bleed. If it does begin to bleed, do not worry, it will stop very quickly.

Pat the skin and the stoma dry with dry wipes. <u>Do not use towels, paper towel, tissue or cotton wool</u> to do this. Towels may carry germs that could infect any areas of the stoma that are bleeding. Cotton wool is too fluffy and may leave fragments sticking to the Stoma. Paper towels and tissues may also leave remnants.

Next, apply a "barrier cream wipe" or stoma paste if that is what you are using. These help protect your skin, while the stoma paste fills in any natural grooves that may affect the adhesion to the skin. If you are subject to bleeding, you may wish to apply some dry antiseptic powder to the affected area.

Now, fit your clean appliance: Take your bag (for single piece appliances), or flange (for two piece appliances) Carefully, bring the bottom edge of the stoma hole adhesive in line with the bottom of your stoma, use a small hand mirror if necessary (as you get more practice the mirror will become redundant). Gently press it into place starting at the bottom and work up being careful to avoid any wrinkles in the flange or bag adhesive.

- If you have problems with leakages or bags bursting, you can try adding a seal that fits around the stoma before applying the bag. The best I have found are hydrocolloid seals by Pelican Healthcare and Eakin. External security seals that fit around the edge of the bag also work very well. I prefer the second nature collection "SecuPlast Seals SP45" and of all else fails, sometimes use the SecuPlast Hydro SPH1. Bullen's Healthcare also makes a great flange tape for specific areas that are prone to leak.

- At this point, you can add odour control or congealing powders through the bottom opening of the bag. If you pop these into the bag beforehand, you may displace some of the powder that will attach itself to the bag adhesive breaking the seal.

- If you are using a one-piece system or a drainable bag, make sure that the pouch is closed securely.

- If using a two-piece system you will now need to clip on the bag to the flange base. Again, work the appliance onto the flange carefully from bottom to top. Once on, check it is firmly in place by giving the bag a gentle tug.

Unwanted Baggage

- To dispose of the soiled bag simply place it with all used wipes etc. in a disposal bag (again provided by the supply companies). If you do not have any disposal bags, you can wrap waste material in a few layers of newspaper, and discard with household waste.

- Check with your local council as to their correct preferred disposal method. Some councils will issue you with a yellow medical waste bin; others accept disposal bags with general household waste.

- Tommy Tippee makes scented nappy disposal bags that can be used in conjunction with a *Tommy Tippee* small sized sealed nappy bin, available from **Mothercare** (prices vary). These are particularly useful for flats where waste has to be carried to another floor/disposal chute as they can remain in the bin for several days without undue odour. **Brabantia** also make a stainless steel bathroom bin but it will only hold two bags at any one time and is much more expensive.

- Do not <u>under any circumstances</u> attempt to flush pouches, flanges or wipes down the toilet, unless the manufacture states the appliance is flushable. Being plastic and solid, they will soon block up the drainage system.

If you have to change your bag away from home, try to find a disabled toilet where there is a sink and clinical waste bin. The additional benefit to using a disabled toilet is that it is generally cleaner than a conventional public toilet due to key-access only and has a sink within reach of the toilet. A special key that fits all public disabled toilets is obtainable VAT and postage free for £3.50 only from **RADAR** at: **www.radar.org.uk** RADAR is a charity and charges for any items on their website are reflected as such. However, be warned - do not put RADAR or RADAR KEY into a search engine as there are many rip-off sites selling RADAR keys at higher prices + VAT + delivery. RADAR keys also appear on ebay and other auction sites at inflated prices and added postage costs; it is a disgraceful way of obtaining money from a vulnerable community!

- A soiled pouch is classed the same as a dirty nappy or used sanitary towel. If you find it necessary to change in an ordinary public toilet, it is perfectly acceptable for ladies to place any soiled appliance or wipes etc. in the sanitary towel bin. Men can place any soiled material in the waste disposal bin, wrapped in paper towel (if available) or toilet paper if not.

- Andrex have just produced a new small emergency mini toilet roll – 50 sheets, available from most supermarkets. This will fit into a pocket or handbag discreetly and is handy, as so many public toilets seem to run out of toilet paper – for ostomates this is an essential carry item!

- Once you are finished, make sure you wash your hands thoroughly and return all unused items to your container or travel bag and stock up if supplies are getting low.

Unwanted Baggage

Emergency Changes

When you are eventually back on your feet and feeling fit, you may want to venture out more often. If you intend to leave the house, it is best to take a small travel bag emergency kit. All of the supply companies provide small carrying cases, dry and wet wipes, water sprays and waste bags as complimentary items. These are especially designed to carry ostomy supplies and will fit into a large handbag or glove compartment of a car.

When travelling, a "bum bag" is a good alternative to hold supplies for both men and women. Gentlemen may also carry a small spare kit in their pockets. There are also some wonderful underpants for men called ***smuggling duds***, which contain a small-buttoned pocket on the front. While this was originally intended to carry condoms, we have had it tested under "clubbing" conditions and it will easily hold a spare bag and a cleansing sachet. For more information, contact: **www.smugglingduds.com**

If you are just nipping into town and back or intend on being out of the house for only an hour you can check your appliance before leaving the house, but **always, *always* take your kit with you**. Accidents can happen when you least expect it!! Your travel kit for two changes should ideally contain:

- Two pouches
- Cleansing gel (in case there is no running water supply) or wipes
- Wet wipes (at least five) in a plastic bag

- Dry wipes (at least five) in a plastic bag

- Aerosol adhesive remover (or you can manage with three or four sachets to save on space)

- Three sachets of barrier wipes

- Two waste bags.

- Odour gel/powder for pouch

- Scissors

- A clothes peg (to clip your clothes out of the way to allow arms-free changing).

If by chance you are caught out without your kit, some pharmacies carry these items. You can also substitute – baby wipes for wet wipes, kitchen towel for dry wipes, plastic freezer bags for disposal bags. Some pharmacies may even carry ostomy bags of some description, but most do not. In extreme desperation, you can manage with a rubber glove held in place by medical tape, plasters or even duct tape available from any general store or pharmacy. Pad with kitchen towel and tape over. If you are not far from home, a sanitary pad or cotton wadding held in place by tape will absorb a small amount of waste. As you gain confidence with your stoma , you will learn the limits of how long you can leave a bag on, how full it can be before problems arise etc.

All of the support associations produce laminated "need to use the toilet" cards. With these, you can go into any large store or restaurant/cafe and producing the card, ask to use their staff toilet facilities. It explains briefly that you have a chronic condition for which you need to use

Unwanted Baggage

a toilet in am emergency. The staff would probably have to check with the Manager beforehand but they hardly ever refuse.

Some of the most common problems can be easily overcome, but some may take time and experimentation. Try not to get downhearted as accidents happen – these are all part of learning to live with a bag. If you are travelling in the UK and a serious problem arises, then go straight to the nearest A&E. If you need to locate a medical facility or pharmacy urgently text "A&E" or "Pharmacy", on a mobile phone to 61121 . This will return a text message with clear directions to your nearest facility.

You may experience initial or occasional problems with your bag. It may burst or leak seemingly without reason but quite often because you have rushed the process of replacing the bag. It is very important to clean the stoma area properly, make sure the area is completely dry, apply a good barrier solution and then apply the bag, holding it in tightly in position by pressing down on the whole area for several minutes.

If you do experience frequent leaking during the night, there is a wonderful new gadget that has just been developed. It is called a "**Stoma Alert"** and clips on to your bag, with the alarm wire fitted to your nightwear. If the bag suddenly expands or movement of liquid is detected then the alarm sounds. It is audible without being offensive and serves to jolt the wearer into action before bedding becomes sodden. A vibrating alternative is available on request. Ileostomates are more prone to leakage that colostomates and urostomates due to the higher liquid output from the stoma. The alarm is not suitable for people with pacemakers. The Stoma Alert is available from:

Nikris ltd
Telephone: 01926 815518 email: info@stomalert.co
www.stomalarm.co.uk

Chapter Seven
Problem Areas
...How to recognise and deal with potential problems quickly.

The following advice is intended only as a general guide. As always, if you are in any doubt <u>whatsoever</u> over your state of health, your stoma or the condition of your skin you should seek medical advice. Some of the more common problems that may arise and helpful ideas are as follows: However, they do not substitute for professional, medical advice.

Dehydration

Dehydration is a common and regular problem for all ostomates. It can quickly become severe and, if neglected, may need a radical solution – hospitalisation! The symptoms of dehydration may include some or any one of the following:

- Dry mouth,
- Dry lips
- Dry or itchy eyes
- Dry skin with a lack of elasticity
- Sunken features, particularly the eyes

- Cold or clammy hands and feet
- Mild headaches,
- A feeling of light-headedness
- Feeling faint or dizzy
- A feeling of exhaustion or tiredness
- Feeling confused or irritable
- A loss of appetite
- A slight burning sensation in your stomach
- A slight feeling of hunger/emptiness
- Itchiness
- Abdominal pain
- Low urine output
- Concentrated, dark urine with a strong odour

If you are dehydrated, this means that you will have lost sugar, salts and minerals, as well as water. You should therefore drink a re-hydration solution that contains all the essential ingredients that you need to re-establish the right balance of body fluids. There are several different re-hydration products available on prescription. If you are at all concerned, immediately consult your GP or pharmacist for advice.

Drinking too much plain water when you are dehydrated can make the problem worse because it can dilute the

Unwanted Baggage

minerals, salts and sugars in your body. A sweet drink, such as a sweet soda (not "diet"), especially Lucozade or an electrolyte drink can replace vital salts.

If you are severely dehydrated, hospitalisation may be required. Additional fluid may be given through a nasogastric tube (up the nose) or saline drip (infusion into a vein).

As one who had had to be hospitalised for rehydration on several occasions, I would add that dehydration can happen very quickly and suggest constant monitoring, by means of regular monthly blood tests, to check levels, that your GP or district nurse can schedule for you.

Leakage

There are several reasons for bag leaks as a new stoma is prone to changes over several months until it settles down. Thereafter, it will change with age and your weight. It will change in size and convexity – it can protrude or sink below the surface of the skin, so different bags should be utilised as the stoma changes.

In each box of bags, there is usually a stoma size guide. At least once a week, place the template over the stoma, excluding any red areas surrounding it. Check that it is the same size. If not, do not hesitate to call your supplier to order a new size. (If it is a standard stock cut-out there will be matching stock number that you can find on the website or discuss this with the call centre). You can also provide an updated template of the required size if it is not. Manufacturers fully understand that bag sizes change during the life of your stoma. You should not return any unused bags as the NHS or the manufacturers will merely throw them away. For health reasons, they may not re-use any stock in opened boxes. If you wish, you can donate them to the various overseas charities mentioned before.

Even with today's advances in stoma care products, all ostomists will admit that leakages happen occasionally. They are a huge source of irritation, not only to the ostomist's pride, but also more importantly to their skin.

If leakage is constant, your skin will become inflamed as waste matter (ileostomates/colostomates) or urine (urostomates) forces its way past the adhesive and is exposed to skin. Initially ensure that you are using the correct shaped bag. Your stoma may have retracted in which case you may need to try a convex bag. Pelican make an excellent range of convex bags and will send samples upon request.

Urostomates will also experience basic leakage problems if the bag is not emptied frequently or if they have problems with the seal due to retraction of the stoma.

If changing the type or manufacturer of the bag does not work, you can try any of the following methods to prevent leakage:

1. Thoroughly cleanse the area around the stoma. Apply a barrier lotion/spray/cream to the area that will be covered by the bag's flange. Wait for it to dry (covering the stoma

Unwanted Baggage

so that it does not leak onto the area) and apply a new bag. Cavilon barrier spray by 3M is one of the best.

2. If the leakage continues, you may want to apply an internal ring/seal that you stick around the stoma before you apply the bag. If you prefer you can apply an external seal after the bag is in position. These seals will keep the bag firmly in place. Internal seals manufactured by Pelican are the most comfortable; Second Seal by Salts is a good external seal. You can use both external and internal seals for maximum protection.

3. Having tried methods 1 & 2 and the stoma continues to leak through the seals, a last resort is a paste solution, manufactured by Eakin. The paste is applied to the skin where the bag will sit. You must wear latex gloves to apply this paste, which is very difficult to remove, and leave the bag on for 48 hours after application. Use a citrus adhesive remover sachet from Pelican to remove the paste.

Do consult your stoma nurse throughout the above procedures. It is important to keep her informed of any problems you are having and allow her to suggest other methods.

If leakage only occurs after you have been bending or stretching, you are creasing the flange that will cause leakages. You may benefit from wearing a small security belt. The major ostomy manufacturers all produce a stoma belts and caps. Wear the cap over the pouch, and secure it in place with the belt.

Leakage can also be caused by constant diarrhoea. You are more likely to experience diarrhoea if you have had an ileostomy. If you have had a colostomy, then diarrhoea only becomes prevalent if you have a reaction to certain foods. Trial and error eating will narrow down the culprit! Unfortunately, constant diarrhoea will eventually cause seepage underneath a weak flange or bag, forcing its way out of the sides and base of the bag.

If this happens regularly, your stoma nurse may recommend a course of Loperamide (trade name Imodium), which is available from your GP. Alternatively, you may wish to try 20gm of either Jelly Babies or Marshmallows per day - the gelatine content helps to congeal the pouch content and acts the same way as loperamide. As most ileostomates are prone to a higher liquid output, then a powder or gel sachet placed in a clean bag will clot the contents and prevent leakage.

Standard cosmetic body creams can do more harm than good. You should make sure than any creams or lotions you apply to your skin near the stoma are especially for ostomy requirements (so that they do not stop the bag's adhesion to the skin). Your skin must be clean and dry before you stick the flange on, otherwise the adhesion of the flange to the body will be compromised and result in leakage.

Leakage will also occur if there is a build-up of faecal matter around the stoma (**pancaking**). To prevent pancaking, screw up a piece of toilet tissue and put this in the bottom of the pouch. This will expand the bag, allowing thicker matter to descend. Instead you can add ostozyme lubricating gel or powder (available on prescription), into a clean pouch before application and you will find this reduces pancaking tremendously. A few drops of baby oil also help matter to descend in the bag away from the stoma opening.

Stoma Bridges hold the bag slightly elevated to ensure contents are passed down the bag rather than accumulating (pancaking), around the stoma. They are quite difficult to place properly (immediately near the bag's opening) but once the knack has been acquired, these are effective.

If you gain or lose weight, this can cause the layout of a stoma to change by creating creases in the skin where the less flexible adhesives struggle to stick. Try sucking in your tummy before sticking the flange down.

Sore Skin

If you find the skin around your stoma is sore and there has been no apparent leakage, you may be allergic to the adhesive on the bag you are currently using – change the manufacturer. Alternatively, by using two-piece bags you will also reduce the number of times you have to change the base plate that will rest the skin between changes.

In general, removing the bag more than usual can cause extreme soreness. Any more than three times in twenty-four hours will cause inflammation. Closed or disposable bags are not a good idea in this case. Ideally, change a one-piece bag once a day, either early morning before breakfast or late in the evening, at least three/four hours after a meal.

In all cases of sore skin, careful preparation of the stoma site upon changing is important. The best method is as follows:

- First, put the clean bag to warm on top of a radiator or inside an airing cupboard or use a hairdryer on it for a few minutes and, failing all else, sit on the new bag (with cover attached) while you are removing the old one. These methods will raise the temperature of the adhesive, making it tackier and easier to apply.

- Remove the existing bag carefully using an aerosol adhesive remover. I have found "Appeel No Sting" medical adhesive remover to be one of the best. Gently spray at the edges and hold skin down to remove slowly.

- Remove excess matter with a dry wipe.

- Remove the old adhesive with an adhesive remover wipe such as "appeal no sting" sachets. If you have a particularly strong adhesive, or used an additional paste, then Pelican's citrus adhesive remover will be more effective.

Using a dry wipe rinsed in warm water (soap is optional), clean the stoma thoroughly. If water is not available, use a wet wipe or cleansing gel.

- Dry the area thoroughly with a dry wipe.

- Apply a barrier film – my personal favourite is "LBF no sting barrier" sachet followed by "3M Cavilon spray" barrier, allowing each barrier to dry for at least 30 seconds in turn.

- Apply a very small amount of Ostoseal aloe vera protective powder (or similar ostomate powder) to the irritated parts. Use a cotton bud to apply to the affected area.

When you take a shower, remove the bag altogether to give your skin a rest. If you prefer a bath, apply a small shower "cap" to the stoma as its smaller adhesive area allows water to reach most of the surrounding skin. A Dansac "mini-cap" does the job perfectly and lets you soak and deep clean the sore skin round the stoma.

Do note use bath creams or oils in bath water, as they will leave an oily film around the stoma preventing good adhesion.

No content in the bag

If the bag remains empty for more than five hours after any meal and you are experiencing severe abdominal pain – seek medical advice **immediately**, you may have a blockage. Many ordinary foods can cause blockages, but chewing food properly usually prevents this. Foods to be avoided specifically are nuts, sweet corn and vegetable skins (see listings under the chapter 11).

Bleeding around the stoma

In most cases, this is caused by the flange fitting too tightly, or by cleaning the stoma too vigorously. The stoma has a rich blood source just under the surface that bleeds very easily. However, any bleeding will soon stop and is perfectly normal. Press a gauze pad over the area until it stops and then apply the bag as normal.

However, if you find blood **inside the bag** that has come from inside the body and not from the skin around the stoma you should seek medical advice **immediately**.

If you are undergoing a course of chemotherapy or radiotherapy, these treatments make the stoma very fragile and bleeding will be frequent at every bag change. Apply gentle pressure on the stoma, using a dry wipe and it will soon stop.

Prolapse

A Prolapse may occur in any type of stoma but are more prevalent in loop colostomies and ileostomies. The muscles holding the stoma weaken and allow the bowel to telescope out, increasing the length of the stoma, sometimes by several inches.

A prolapse is not normally painful and will not prevent the stoma functioning but in all instances, you should contact your stoma nurse as soon as possible to examine possible remedies. Surgery may be needed in cases of an extreme prolapsed.

Parastomal hernia

When a stoma is brought to the surface of the abdomen it must pass through the muscles of the abdominal wall, thus a potential site of weakness is created. In the ideal situation, the abdominal wall muscles form a snug fit around the stoma opening.

However, sometimes the muscles come away from the edges of the stoma thus creating a "hernia" which is a protrusion of bowel underneath the stoma incision causing a visible swelling or bulge. It is far more common colostomates than other ostomates.

Factors that can contribute to causing a stomal hernia to occur include extreme coughing or sneezing, putting on too much weight, weight-lifting, stretching or an infection in the wound at the time the stoma was made.

The development of a stomal hernia is often a gradual phenomenon, with the area next to the stoma stretching and becoming weaker with the passage of time. This weakness, or gap, means that every time you strain, cough, sneeze or even stand up, the area of the abdomen next to the stoma bulges, or the whole stoma itself protrudes as the rest of the abdominal contents behind it push it forwards.

As with all hernias, the size will increase as time goes by. Stoma hernias are rarely painful, but are usually uncomfortable and can become extremely inconvenient.

There are surgeons who advocate that small stoma hernias that are not causing any discomfort do not need any treatment other than wearing a wide, firm colostomy/ileostomy belt. This is probably true with small hernias in people who are very elderly and infirm or for people for whom an anaesthetic would be dangerous (serious heart or breathing problems, for example).

However, for most people, operative repair of the stoma hernia should be given serious consideration to improve the quality of life, and to prevent progressive enlargement of the hernia with time and make it easier to manage the daily maintenance of the bag and stoma.

A hernia makes it difficult for pouches to work effectively especially in creating a complete seal to keep faecal matter (or urine) off the skin. The position of the stoma can be altered by a parastomal hernia increasing the stoma's size making it more difficult to see. This large bulge under clothing can be very embarrassing.

Retracted Stoma

A retracted stoma is one that has sunk below skin level, almost resembling a belly button. A retraction may be partially or completely below the skin level.

This can be due to a technical difficulty at the time of surgery that may emerge over time; any weight gain or loss post-operatively; or during pregnancy when the stoma may become stretched.

Retraction may cause leakage and skin irritation problems as it can often be difficult to obtain a good seal around the retracted stoma.

It is important to seek advice from your stoma nurse who may refer you back to your consultant. In extreme cases, surgical reconstruction or refashioning of the stoma may have to be done.

Major skin problems

Ulcers, bruising and pressure sores may arise from trauma from a pouch or belt that supports a pouch. Non-ambulatory patients seem to be more prone to pressure sores in the abdominal area.

The misuse of convex stoma products has also been associated with pressure sores, ulcers and peri-stomal bruising. Ask advice from your stoma nurse if you notice any of these occurring.

Rectal issues

Removal of the rectum:

In many ostomy cases, the rectum is also removed. In the early days after your operation, you may experience pain specifically in the rectal area for which painkillers will be given. The pain will improve in time but painkillers are often needed for the first three months after surgery.

You may also find that you will not be able to sit comfortably for long periods of time post-operatively, but getting up and walking around will relieve the pressure from your perineal area. Intercourse may also prove painful for a few months until the external wound site has healed properly.

It is very important to check with your GP or stoma nurse as to when you can resume intercourse after rectum removal.

Rectal spasms (when the rectum has not been removed)

In some cases following a colostomy or ileostomy, a rectal stump is left in place. Experiences of rectal sensations are then quite common, especially shortly after surgery. These can be quite painful and frightening. You should sit on the toilet for a few minutes and may pass a small amount of mucus. Again, this is normal and the sensation will pass. After a couple of months these feelings should stop.

If you are at all worried, do talk to your stoma nurse who may ask your GP to prescribe Buscopan (or similar) that will calm the rectum and a pain medication if necessary. If symptoms continue after the first six months, you should make an appointment with your consultant. Further surgery may be necessary to remove the rectum in its entirety.

Sex

Please see the chapter on intimacy for sexually related issues

Odour

"Do I smell?" – is a common question for most new ostomates. The simple answer is "no", but there are times when odour *may* become a problem.

When you change the bag, you will notice some odour. The smell is normal, but may be more intense or simply different, dependent upon which type of food you have eaten. Most suppliers will provide a spray for the toilet that will mask residual odours.

Odour emanating from the bag area can be caused by a leakage and is a first warning sign of an accident about to happen. Odour can also be cause by wind. There is a small filter hole at the top of any bag and, if there is a build-up of wind, then it will escape, with an accompanying odour through this filter. To minimise this odour, you can cover the filter with the stickers provided inside the box of bags. For colostomates and ileostomates, the filter is there to prevent a build-up of wind in the bag; so, if you cover the filter, make sure you empty the bag more frequently or it could burst. Excessive wind will be caused by and during air-travel due to cabin pressure, so make sure that you examine your bag at regular intervals during a flight. Wind is caused by different foods – see the chapter 11 on diet for a full list of "windy foods"!

Scuba diving can also cause a massive build-up of wind. Most divers try to time their dives to four hours after a meal and always empty their bag just before beginning a dive.

For urostomates, a smell of urine is only a problem if the outside of the bag is not cleaned at the emptying site. Splash back contributes to this, so empty the bag slowly and carefully. Ensure the bag is properly dried after re-sealing. Certain foods such as asparagus and fish can make urine smell but this should be contained by the bag.

If you think you can still smell an unpleasant aroma, there are many sprays, odour absorbing gels, tablets and powders that you can insert into the bag, before application. All of these are available on prescription. Do not use any perfumed spray or cream that is not specifically designed for the bag as ostomy products are uniquely designed to prevent damage to the bag or your skin.

You may imagine that you can smell the bag. This is very common, but in most cases unfounded. It is the bag content that smells, not you! The bag can quite adequately contain the smell provided it is emptied frequently and the edges cleaned upon discharge. To be completely reassured about an odour problem, ask someone else if they can smell anything.

Unwanted Baggage

Bathing and swimming

You may bathe, shower, swim or use a Jacuzzi with a bag. You can shower (not bathe or swim obviously), without your pouch if you wish, normal exposure to air, or water will not harm the stoma, Water cannot enter the ostomy opening.

Most people however prefer to leave the pouch on while washing or you can use a mini pouch (DANSAC mini-cap) which I find more comfortable. However, if swimming or using a Jacuzzi, there are simple guidelines to follow:

- If you are worried about the bag slipping, you can protect the bag's edge with an additional flange or micro pore waterproof tape available from any good pharmacy. You can also wear a waterproof bag cover from www.bullens.com

- You can purchase a specially designed ostomy swimsuit from

    www.whiterosecollection.com
    www.vblush.com
    www.ostomart.co.uk
    www.cui.co.uk

- **Marks and Spencer**'s also offer tankini style regular costumes with longer tops and short-style bottoms. These can quite adequately cover a bag at much more affordable pricing than the specialised garments.

- Male ostomates may wish to wear an additional support garment sold in most sports shops.

- For men with a stoma above the waistline, or if you feel self-conscious about the scars, you may wish to swim in a tank top or t-shirt.

- Eat lightly and empty the pouch before any water based sport..

- For sanitary reasons you should always wear a pouch when you go swimming.

Prescription medicines

All time-release medication, birth control pills and some other tablets may pass through directly into the bag without entering your system. They are therefore, **ineffective**. Ask your GP or pharmacist to change time-release medication to regular tablets or a liquid or patch form of your medication. Ask him to check all your medication for its absorption factors as other coated medications may not be wholly absorbed and pass into the bag. You can also check the bag for any remnants of tablets.

You should especially re-evaluate birth control methods as the pill is proven ineffective following a colostomy or ileostomy. (See the chapter on pregnancy).

Unwanted Baggage

Serious issues

If you suffer any of the following problems**, it is essential that you contact your GP or stoma nurse as soon as possible**. If for any reason, you are unable to contact either of them for more than twelve hours after you notice these symptoms, then visit your nearest A & E.

- Severe cramps or abdominal pain that lasts more than three hours.
- Unusually strong odour for more than twenty-four hours (if you have not eaten any contributory foods).

Any dramatic or unusual changes in the appearance of your stoma ; any swelling in particular.

- Any obstruction of the stoma. An indication of this is that the bag remains empty of slightly full with liquid only after six hours, providing you have eaten normally. A prolonged obstruction will also cause severe pain.

Any signs of a prolapse of the stoma.

- Discharge on the surface of the stoma that is not from the stoma opening.
- Lumps appearing in the skin near to the stoma (fistulas).

Any visible narrowing or closing of the stoma spout

- (stenosis).

- Visible pus oozing from the stoma or present in the bag

- Bleeding from the stoma opening or any amount of blood in the pouch. *(Note: Eating beetroot will lead to blood-like colouration in the pouch).

- Severe injury or cut to the stoma.

- Continuous bleeding between the stoma and the skin.

- Watery/liquid discharge lasting more than five or six hours.

- Chronic and constant skin irritation unresolved by change of bag manufacturer or the application of soothing creams.

- Small holes that may appear on or around the stoma, discharging faecal matter in addition to the stoma "spout".

Note: If for any reason you are hospitalised again, make sure you take your ostomy supplies with you, as the hospital may not have you preferred brand.

Chapter Eight
Hints and Tips
...A Few Ideas and Suggestions to Assist New Ostomates

- If you are changing a bag with your clothes on, roll up your shirt/sweater/dress etc. at the front to reveal the ostomy. Take a **clothes peg** and peg the clothes out of the way. This way you have both hands free to clean your ostomy, and not have to struggle with one hand as the other holds your clothes up. You can also use the clothes peg when emptying the bag a well. A single clothes peg will easily fit into a pocket.

- If you live in a flat or apartment with waste disposal facilities several floors away or if you are at all concerned about the temporary disposal of waste bags etc There are specially designed bins available from (prices may vary from time to time):

    Mothercare called the **Tommy Tippee** bin. It has a vacuum seal to contain all odours and will hold at least five disposal bags. (It was originally designed for waste nappies but is ideal for ostomate use.) The cost is £9.99 and spare liner bags can be purchased although plastic carrier bags work just as well.

Angelcare Nappy disposal System is available on amazon (www.amazon.co.uk) at £7.49 information available on www.angelcare-uk.co.uk

Brabantia also make a seal bathroom bin.

- Incense and scented candles in the bathroom help with odour problems.

- If you wear your bag in the shower or bath and do not need to change it, wear a waterproof cover and use a hair dryer to dry the bag.

- A baby's waterproof bib around the neck of the bag will keep a wet bag from lying onto skin while you are drying the rest of you.

- Waterproof over-bags can be obtained on prescription from Bullen's healthcare. **www.bullens.com**

- Keep your supplies organised – set aside an area of a bathroom closet for ostomy equipment or use plastic/wicker container boxes. This will also help you to note the amount of supplies you have on hand and when you need to re-order.

- Keep a list of regular products by the phone with the phone number of your supplier. Try to order a month's worth of products at a time. If you are not going to be at home to accept the deliveries, ask your supplier to leave the package in a convenient place or with a neighbour. Note all holiday delivery times to ensure continuity

Unwanted Baggage

of supply. Make sure your supplier marks the package "No signature required".

- To help the waste empty from your pouch easier, spray the inside of the pouch with a vegetable cooking spray or add a few drops of baby oil – before applying the bag. Both of these help prevent pancaking as well.

- Showering on a regular basis without your appliance on is soothing and very good for your skin. Take a small gauze pad with you to contain faecal matter in place as you dry.

- Cloth bag covers prevent skin irritation on your abdomen and legs from the bag. You can either make these or order them made-to-measure (on prescription), from **www.bullens.com** or, **www.ostomart.co.uk** . There are also a few private manufacturers but these are not available on prescription – bag covers from them cost £9-£15 each in the UK and $15-$30 each from the US plus postage from both. See Chapter 14 for suppliers.

- Free prescription underwear can be ordered from **www.cuiwear.com** (6 pairs per year, limited styles/material only.)

- Disposable underwear is essential if you are travelling for long distances or going into hospital. Available from **www.thebowelmovement.co.uk**

- Waste matter builds up while you are sleeping. To avoid "pancaking" insert a stoma bridge made by **www.*opus-healthcare.co.uk***

- To avoid splashing when emptying the bag, throw a wad of toilet paper in the front of the toilet bowl, this will stop liquid matter bouncing back.

- For a 'clean' feeling after emptying your pouch, obtain some 60ml syringes from your local pharmacy (usually a small fee). Fill the syringe with water and insert into the neck of the pouch. Empty the water into the pouch and have a good rinse around. Drain the water away and dry the neck by wrapping toilet tissue around a finger.

- Carry a spare mattress pad to change in a car, protect the seat etc.

- Carry some disposable /spare underwear at all times. After one distressing incident, I always carry a complete change of clothes when leaving the house.

- Paper disposable toilet seat covers are great for travelling. Available in three packs of ten covers at **www.cleanseatuk.com** (they also supply disposable toileting systems such as "traveljohn" for travelling).

Chapter Nine
Irrigation
...A Viable Alternative?

Irrigation is not possible for ileostomists or urostomists.

Irrigation is only possible for **_some_** colostomists. Irrigation consists of giving your bowel a washout or enema through the stoma instead of wearing and emptying a bag. A plug, cap or even a mini bag can be worn over the stoma between irrigation procedures to prevent any leakage. .

Both your surgeon and stoma nurse must approve this procedure. They will also advise on whether it may be required daily, or on alternate days. An irrigation procedure takes about three quarters of an hour, but it is still worthwhile if you have the time and patience.

Initially your stoma nurse will guide you through the irrigation process and will supply you with the equipment required for each irrigation:-

- A water bag, complete with hose and cone.
- Plastic sleeves.
- Sheets of wipes.
- Disposable bags, caps and plugs.

You will also need a few additional extras from around the house:-

- A means of hanging up the water bag - a fixed hook, metal meat hook, string, firm shower rail window catch etc. approx. just above head height and within easy reach.
- A plastic indoor or child's watering can.
- A wooden spring clothes peg.
- Absorbent toilet paper.
- Matches/air freshener

The plastic see-through water bag is rather like a hot water bottle in shape and has a handle with which to hang it. It will hold four pints of water at blood heat. Some suppliers make these water bags with a built-in thermometer which helps ensure that the water temperature is just right at 37C (98.4F).

Attached to the base of the bag is a hose approx.120cms. long with a plastic cone at the end and a control switch. The open-ended plastic sleeve has an adhesive ring near the top that sticks over the stoma .

Preparation:

- Ensure the bathroom temperature is comfortable and that you have all the equipment you need to hand.

Unwanted Baggage

- Most people irrigate sitting on the loo, but it can be easier to lie on a towel in an empty bath with a cushion.

- Having chosen your position, fix the empty water bag securely above head height using a strong hook. A length of string can be useful for fine adjustments. The head of water is necessary to penetrate your inner reaches. Hang the bag on the hook.

- Using the water can, fill the suspended bag full with water from the hot tap, then add enough water from the cold tap until the correct temperature is reached (37C/98.4F). If using a bag with a built-in thermometer, you can easily see the green indicator moving down the scale. Approx 4 pints are needed to complete the irrigation.

- Now for irrigating, Strip off the old bag, cap or plug. Stick the sleeve over your stoma , settle into a comfortable position with the end of the sleeve hanging between your legs and down into the toilet bowl (or in the direction of the bath plughole).

- Place the cone into the stoma through the top of the sleeve and start the control to allow water into the bowel, making sure the water goes into the bowel and not straight down the sleeve. You must ensure that the displaced air can escape. This procedure takes about five minutes. Sometimes the peristalsis of the bowel (involuntary muscular movement), which pushes the waste material along the colon, kicks into action so patience is required.

- The flow-back starts almost immediately, so be ready with a full watering can, to pour water down the inside of the sleeve to reduce the smell and direct the waste away rapidly. If you are in the bath, quickly fold the bottom of the sleeve to the top, peg into place and move over to the bowl for the rapid evacuation of the bowel. You can do this standing or sitting. For your own comfort, keep the watering can at the ready to wash down each flood of faeces.

- Normally this phase is the busiest part of the procedure. You will notice that at first there will be very small stool formation but very soon it will become totally without form – like wet mud apart from tiny bits of undigested food e.g. sweet corn etc. This stage of irrigation ends with a gurgle and explosive splatter. This is an indication that the bowel is empty and very soon you will be able to put on the cap, plug or cover. For the next twenty-three hours, you will then be able to forget you even have a colostomy.

- Finally: The cleaning process. There may be a slight odour in the room. Use an air freshener, or open a window. This should clear will the air. Put the equipment away, remembering to wash out the water bag thoroughly and

Unwanted Baggage

dry it afterwards. Dispose of used sleeve and bag etc.

If, after several tries, you find that you are uncomfortable with the procedure, it is not an admission of failure to return to a bag. Many, many colostomists are happier wearing a conventional bag.

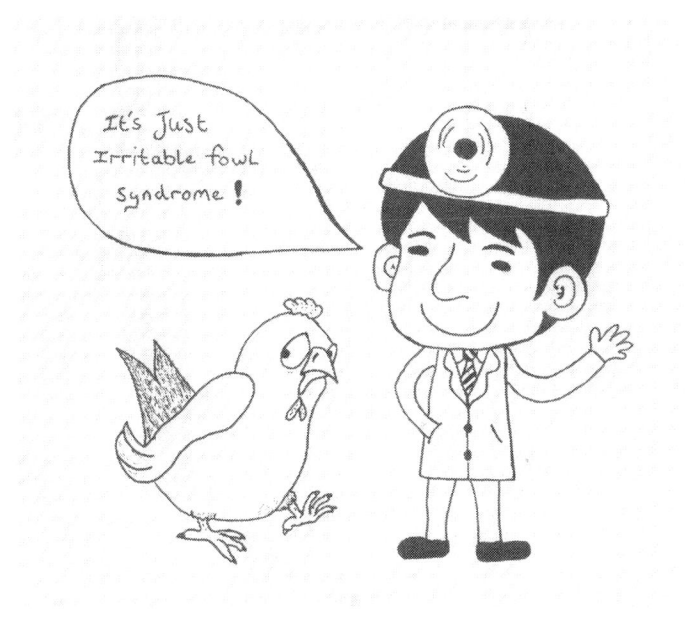

Chapter Ten
A Reversal
...Ostomy Reversal following temporary keyhole surgery.

Ostomy reversal is only possible for temporary colostomy patients.

Due to advances in keyhole surgery, temporary colostomies are becoming more viable. A colostomy reversal, (also referred to as a laparoscopic colostomy reversal), is a surgical procedure in which the large intestine (colon) and rectum are reconnected after a prior, temporary, keyhole colostomy.

Initial surgery is performed by the "keyhole" method, involving a short stay of a few days in hospital. A small section of the bowel is removed and the bowel allowed to 'rest' for a few months. A temporary stoma will be made and a bag has to be worn in the interim.

The reversal surgery will involve another short hospital stay. The new keyhole operation will leave you with two very small scars. The location of these scars depend on the operating Surgeon, but one is usually under the navel and one somewhere else on your belly near the stoma

Unwanted Baggage

area. This is so they can insert their implements and an air-hose into the body. The air hose inflates the abdomen area and lights it so the Surgeon then has some room to manoeuvre whilst operating. Because the wounds are so small and the operation is not too invasive, you will not feel too painful afterwards.

The procedure will be to re-enter the abdominal cavity, usually through the original scar, and cut around the colostomy to free it from the skin and the abdominal wall muscles. The surgeon will then join up the bowel to the remaining rectum either using special stapling instruments or sutures (stitches). This will restore the normal function of the large bowel so that you will return to passing faeces in the normal way. Your wound will be closed with stitches, including the stoma where the colostomy was positioned.

When the bowel has been disconnected from the rectum for some time, the rectum has to readjust to its former pattern. Usually, this means that you may be slightly incontinent for twenty-four hours and may need about a week to return to regular, controlled, bowel movements. Your bowel movements may be loose for some time afterwards.

How long you will be in hospital after the reversal varies from patient to patient and depends on how quickly you recover from the operation and the anaesthetic. Most patients having this type of bowel surgery will be in hospital for seven to ten days.

Time for a full recovery from this surgery varies. It can take up to two or three months. You should consider who is going to look after you during the early part of this time. You may have family or close friends nearby who are able to support you or care for you in your home during the early part of your recovery period. After you return home, you will need to take it easy and should expect to get easily tired to begin with. The district nurse will remove non-dissolving stitches that seal the wound after ten days. If you do not have any help, the hospital will liaise with social services to arrange temporary carers and meals on wheels.

Following a reversal, you should avoid strenuous exercise and lifting for up to twelve weeks. Lighter exercise, such as walking and light housework is encouraged as soon as you feel well enough. You may have some instances of light bowel incontinence so a small pad should be used for the first month until you are confident that this has stopped. If it continues for longer, then consult your GP.

You should not drive until you feel confident that you could perform an emergency stop without discomfort, which could be at least six weeks after your operation. It is your responsibility to check with your insurance company to make sure that you are properly covered under these circumstances.

Most people should not return to work for three months. It depends on:

- How quickly you recover.
- Whether or not your work is physical in any way.

Unwanted Baggage

- Whether of not regular driving is involved beyond commuting to and from work.

- Whether you need any extra treatment after surgery.

Even if you think you feel well enough, it is still essential to check with your GP before returning to work.

Dependent upon the original cause for colostomy, and how your bowel movements proceed in the months following the reversal, you may need a full colostomy later in life. It is sad to say that a high percentage of temporary colostomy patients have to have a permanent colostomy later in life.

Chapter Eleven
A Post Operative Diet Guide
...Diet Guidance for Ostomy Patients

Your gastrointestinal tract is a filter absorbing those things that your body needs. It allows the residuary stool (waste), to pass through. To structure a correct diet it is essential that you know exactly what portions of the bowel have been removed and what remains. Ask your surgeon for these details. If you have been unable to track down the information upon discharge, you can ask you Stoma Nurse, as she will have these details. Your nutritional needs are based upon the extent of the bowel remaining. Ostomy surgery requires that you eat a regular balanced diet that includes the necessary vitamins, minerals and calories.

If you have had a long history of bowel disease, multi-vitamin supplements are essential, dependent upon regular blood test results. Your GP will prescribe these based on these findings.

Eating is important. It is essential to eat at regular intervals, Missing a meal will increase the incidence of watery stools and wind. If you go for several hours without eating and then consume a full meal, you may find you suffer a "stoma rush" – a rather sudden surge

Unwanted Baggage

into the bag that can cause leakage and may feel painful. Avoid fasting at al costs. A proper balanced diet helps to improve the bag's function. You will also sleep better by limiting foods in the late evening. When you have had part of your intestine removed, your body will not absorb all the nutrition you need to maintain health. Therefore, you actually need to eat more than you used to and re-think your diet. Be warned, it goes against most "healthy diet teachings

St Mark's hospital for intestinal and colorectal disorders in London advises the following extract from its Dieticians handouts for ostomy patients).

Your diet needs to be
- High in Energy
- High in Fat
- High in Protein
- High in Salt
- Low in Fibre

This means using real butter, full milk, and spreading it thickly. Adding sugar and salt to meals. Spreading Jam, honey thickly on bread or add to porridge, full fat yogurts or milk puddings

- Eating more cakes and biscuits
- Trying dishes made with cream and cheese
- Adding double cream to cereals, hot drinks and soups

- Frying foods such as meat, fish and potatoes.

For further information, contact **St Mark's hospital Department of Clinical Nutrition Tel: 02088692666**

Each day you will loose a lot of salt from your stoma and it is very important to maintain a high-salt diet. If, like me, you have been cutting down on salt for years, then try adding soya sauce, garlic or celery salt or Aromat (Knorr product) to meals instead of pure salt.

If you are concerned about your diet, keep food charts detailing the kind of food, the exact amount and time of consumption (including any snacks) and liquid intake. Do this for about a month and arrange a blood test to include vitamin, potassium, liver function and iron levels. Once the results are in, make an appointment to meet the hospital's dietician. They will examine the chart and compare it with current blood levels indicating any problem areas. This is an essential exercise to ensure you are maintaining the right nutrients.

If you suffer from dehydration on a regular basis, you can make up your own **daily electrolyte mix.** The solution should be made fresh each day. The ingredients are available from most chemists and can be prescribed by a GP.

- 30 ml glucose
- 5 ml sodium chloride
- 2.5 ml sodium bicarbonate

- 1 litre water. – You can add flavouring such as Ribena, orange juice etc. to make it more palatable.

Note: For your GP: The Rx formula is Glucose 20g; sodium chloride 2.5g;sodium bicarbonate 2.5g.

Specifics on nutrients

Lack of vitamins A, B12, C, D and E and potassium are common in patients following bowel or bladder surgery. Vitamin supplements are available in drop or powder form that can be more easily absorbed than tablets or capsules. Very low iron levels (B^{12}) can be topped up by injection or intravenous drip. .The simple monthly blood test will confirm an individual's need for vitamin supplement levels. Ongoing monthly blood tests are essential following bowel or bladder removal. Details of vitamin needs are as follows:

- **Vitamin A** boosts the immune system and is necessary to maintain a healthy mucous membrane in the eye. Lack of vitamin A can cause eye problems. It also plays a role in the body's immune response and in the function of adrenal glands that control the way in which the body responds to stress. There is considerable evidence to show that stress can trigger a flare-up in IBD illnesses, making Vitamin A vital in preventing future incidents.

- **Vitamin B^9 and B^{12}** (also known as folic acid), are essential. A deficient intake of folic acid can impair the maturation of young red blood cells, resulting in folic-acid-deficiency anaemia. Foliate deficiency is believed to contribute to the onset of chronic illnesses.

- **Vitamin C** aids in the alleviation of inflammation and is believed to help prevent the formation of fistulas in Crohn's patients.

- **Vitamin D** maintains healthy bones and cartilage. It also helps the body to absorb calcium. Many Crohn's patients experience bone deterioration making Vitamin D essential. Vitamin D has other roles in human health, including modulation of neuromuscular and immune function and reduction of inflammation.

- **Vitamin E** is an antioxidant. Antioxidants act to protect your cells against the effects of free radicals, which are potentially damaging by-products of energy metabolism. Free radicals can damage cells and may contribute to the development of cardiovascular disease and cancer. Studies are underway to determine whether vitamin E, through its ability to limit production of free radicals, might help prevent or delay the development of those chronic diseases. Vitamin E also plays a role in immune function.

- A good level of **potassium** is essential. All IBD patients are prone to hypokalemia (low potassium), the symptoms of which include weakness, lack of energy, muscle cramps,

Unwanted Baggage

stomach disturbances, an irregular heartbeat, and occasionally, an abnormal EKG reading (electrocardiogram, a test that measures heart function). Good hydration is the key to maintaining potassium levels. However, if hydration levels drop, Hypokalemia may result, caused by the body losing too much potassium through urination. Regular blood tests will reveal low levels and supplements may be prescribed. If supplements do not work, regular outpatient infusions may be needed.

- Your eyes need Lutein (as well as Vitamin A), which can help to prevent potentially blinding conditions such as uveitis and macular degeneration, to which Crohn's patients are susceptible.

Important food hints and tips for colostomists:

- **<u>A limited amount of Fibre rich foods are important only to colostomists</u>**, especially upon release in the period from hospital discharge to six months afterwards. Selections of fibre-rich foods include Potatoes, Spaghetti, Rice, Yams, Leeks, Swedes, Lentils, Sprouts, Carrots, and Spinach.

- Eat at regular intervals - an empty stomach will produce wind.

- Small, frequent meals are recommended.
- Chew all your food thoroughly to reduce stoma blockages.
- One portion daily of potatoes, rice or pasta will reduce the frequency and irritation of stoma activity.
- Drink plenty of fluids – four to six glasses/mugs are recommended for colostomates.
- Avoid excess caffeine.

Important hints and tips for ileosotmists:

- **<u>Avoid High Fibre foods</u>.**
- Eat regularly –an empty stomach will produce wind.
- Small frequent meals are recommended.
- Chew all your food thoroughly to reduce stoma blockages.
- One portion daily of potatoes, rice or pasta will reduce frequency and irritation of stoma activity.
- High potassium foods – yoghurt, fish, bananas, avocados, green beans and beetroot will help control consistency.
- Drink eight glasses/mugs of fluid a day. Reduce this slightly if you have a constant liquid

Unwanted Baggage

output. The thicker the output, the more fluid you can drink. Sweetened (absolutely <u>no diet drinks</u>) sodas, colas and Lucozade are ideal. Water should be consumed together with a salty product such as crisps and sweet products such as plain chocolate; this combination will maintain a good level of glucose and potassium. Chemical sugar substitute products must not be used under any circumstances.

- Avoid as much caffeine as possible

Important hints and tips for Urostomists:

- For Urostomists to maintain a healthy kidney function you should drink sufficient fluids to keep the urine diluted. You can see this easily by the colour of urine in the bag. Ideally, it should be a pale yellow. The darker the urine, the more you should increase fluid intake. However, take into consideration that certain foods can discolour urine and others can create a strong odour.

- Urostomists should also maintain an acid-base (pH) balance. Combine acid-ash with neutral foods. Ideal acid-ash foods include meat, bread, cereals, cheese, crackers, cranberries, eggs, pasta, rice, prunes, plums and fish. Neutral foods include butter, coffee, cream, honey, salad oils, syrups, tapioca and tea.

- Foods to avoid are alkaline-ash foods that include milk, bananas, beans, beetroot, greens, and unfortunately, most other fruits and vegetables contain alkaline ash, however, a moderate consumption of fruit and vegetables will help to maintain vitamin levels. Ask your dietician to advise you based on urine tests.

- Keep a urine PH test kit handy. This will let you know what levels need adjustment, if any.

Colostomists' and Ileostomists' Output

For colostmists and ileostomists, it is important to know the effects that different foods have on faecal output. Use trial and error to determine your individual tolerance. Do not be afraid to try foods that you like, but try smaller amounts at first until you are sure of the resultant output.

If you are worried about your diet, please consult your stoma nurse who will refer you to a hospital dietician.

General guidelines are as follows:

Foods that might obstruct the stoma:

- Apple skins
- Potato skins
- Raw cabbage

Unwanted Baggage

- Lettuce
- Sweet corn
- Popcorn
- Celery
- Coconut
- Dried Fruits
- Whole mushrooms
- Oranges
- Nuts
- Pineapple
- Seeds
- grapes

Foods that produce wind, causing odour or bursting bags:

- Fizzy or carbonated Alcoholic Drinks*

    *You can set these aside once poured and the wait until the bubbles decrease to avoid wind.

- Fizzy or carbonated Non-alcoholic Drinks*

See above.
- Beans
- Soy products
- Cabbage, cooked
- Cauliflower
- Cucumber
- Dairy Products in excess
- Chewing Gum
- Milk in excess
- Onions
- Radishes

Foods that produce intense faecal odour:

- Asparagus
- Baked Beans
- Broccoli
- Cabbage
- Cod Liver Oil
- Eggs
- Fish
- Garlic

Unwanted Baggage

- Onions
- Peanut Butter
- Strong Cheese

Foods that produce normal colour changes:

These are not to be avoided, but these may appear to cause concern due to the change in faecal output.

- Asparagus
- Beetroot
- Food Colours
- Iron Pills
- Liquorice
- Red Jelly
- Strawberries
- Tomato sauces

Foods that can help to relieve blockages*:

- Warm drinks
- Cooked Fruits
- Cooked Vegetables

- Fresh Fruit
- Natural fruit Juices
- One litre of Water, consumed quickly.

*These can occasionally relieve mild blockages. If the bag remains empty for more than six hours, call your stoma nurse of GP.

Foods that may cause an increase in faecal output in colostomists but may cause diarrhoea in ileostomist:

- Alcoholic Beverages
- Whole Grains
- Bran Cereals
- Cooked Cabbage
- Fresh Fruit
- Leafy Green Vegetables
- Milk
- Prunes
- Raisins
- Raw Vegetables
- Spicy Foods

Treat all these with caution, try a small amount to test whether or not these affect you, everyone is different.

Foods that can prevent increased odour:

- Cranberry Juice
- Orange Juice
- Parsley
- Tomato Juice
- Yoghurt

Foods that can control diarrhoea or thicken output:

- Applesauce
- Bananas
- Boiled white Rice
- Tapioca
- Jelly babies
- Marshmallows
- Gelatine products
- Cheese
- White bread

- Pasta
- Pretzels
- Creamy peanut butter (avoid chunky peanut butter as it contains portions of nuts which may block the stoma)

Cookery Books?

There are a number of cookery books written for ostomists but frankly, these are a waste of time. Everybody is so different. IBD patients react differently to food depending upon how much of the colon or bowel remains. Urostomists have lesser concerns with diet but more concerns with liquid input.

Generally, you can eat what you like as long as it is in moderation. Use your favourite recipes, taking into consideration the above guidelines of the affects some foods may have. If you then find that a specific food or drink causes diarrhoea then avoid it as much as possible.

Do not hesitate to ask for an appointment with the hospital dietician to discuss a sensible diet if you have any concerns. These are the only real experts and can design a perfect diet based on all your own medical information and taking into consideration your own personal preferences. There are NO generalisations for ostomists.

For ideas on basics, do have a look at the Chapter on Cooking for an Ostomate, written by my husband, - carer, chief cook and bottle washer.

Home Parenteral Feeding (HPN)

It is important to mention HPN, but I must stress that this is implemented in extreme cases, and only where high output stomas cannot be corrected by diet, medication or any other method. In these cases, a patient might have to begin a special diet administered by tube, known as Parenteral Feeding. This process normally begins in hospital as a boost. However, on some occasions it may be continued at home.

HPN replaces normal food, although in some cases, an occasional small meal may be permitted in agreement with the dietician. An HPN patient must follow the agreed course of HPN treatment and must not add extra conventional food or snacks unless agreed upon beforehand with the dietician.

Any drinks/ancillary fluids must also be agreed upon at the initiation of the course of HPN. Many people who are on HPN are still able to leave their house as it is only during the time of diet administration (normally during the night), that they have to remain in one place. HPN patients are able to travel and enjoy holidays and sports activities. It is always important to maintain a good quality of life at all times. HPN treatment is administered via an infusion bag of between one and five litres of fluid, via a volumetric pump to an in-dwelling intravenous central line in the patient. Generally, patients infuse these nutrients over a limited period (usually 12 hours overnight). At the end of the infusion, the patients can disconnect themselves from the feeding and can then lead an independent existence.

For a small group of patients subcutaneous fluid may be an appropriate option. This form of parenteral fluid and electrolyte provision does not require a central venous catheter.

The content of the feeding bags is variable depending on patient needs, from simple intravenous fluids to entire nutrient requirements including protein, carbohydrates, fat, mineral and trace elements. The feeding bags are compounded in a hospital or commercial pharmacy and are then delivered to patients in their own home. It is customary for patients to have two weeks supply of feed nutrition on hand. The majority of patients are self-caring for their central line and nutrients but many have their nutrients supervised by a family member, carer, or district nurse. For further information contact:

PNNT

www.pnnt.com
Patients on intravenous and naso-gastric Nutrition Therapy
PO Box 3126
Christchurch
Dorset
BH23 2XS

Unwanted Baggage

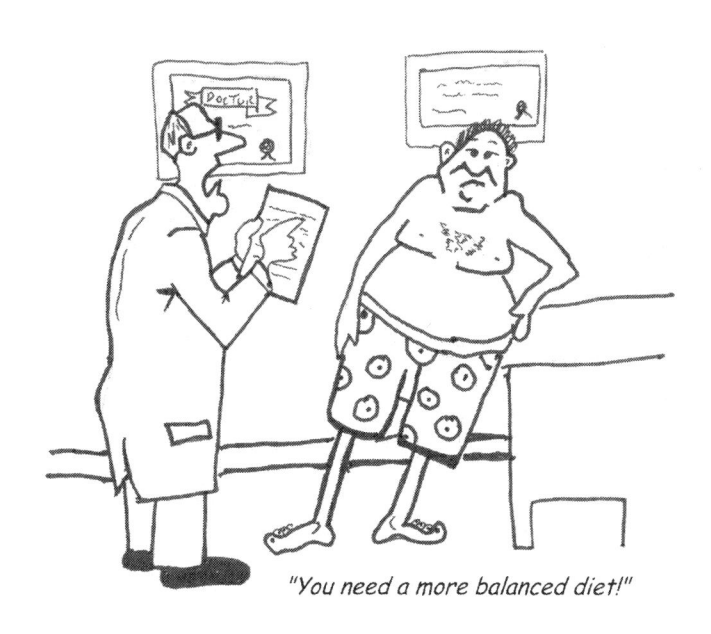

"You need a more balanced diet!"

Chapter Twelve
Exercise & Sports
...Guidelines for Activities

General Guidelines

Three months after any ostomy operation, your body will have adjusted to its internal and external changes. An ostomist should then be able to enjoy most forms of exercise that they did beforehand.

You should however, take medical advice on participating in any extremely rough contact sports or heavy/weight lifting. If you have not participated in sports for a while due to the illness that incurred the stoma, it may be slow going depending on how long you have been out of the game. Gentle exercise is good for any ostomate and a physiotherapist may recommend specific exercises; swimming is by far the best form of exercise, even sitting in a gentle Jacuzzi is excellent therapy. Movement is essential – the amount however, will depend upon both the physical and psychological abilities of the ostomate.

Do not let yourself be pushed into anything you do not want to do or do not feel comfortable about. It is difficult and embarrassing to change in a public or school/work locker room or use an open shower if you are wearing an

Unwanted Baggage

ostomy bag. Fortunately, there are many sports facilities with separate disabled changing facilities.

It is extremely important for young ostomates to be allowed privacy before and after school or club sports. **The school must be apprised of the situation**, and every effort should be made to include the young ostomate in sports sessions.

By law, every School has to arrange for the young ostomate to change or shower in privacy (usually by using a disabled toilet and shower). If a child is excluded from sport, they may feel left out. They may be teased by their classmates.

All aspects of the ostomy must be discussed at length with the school or sports club to ensure maximum integration in as many activities as the child wishes to participate in. If a young ostomate does not want to join in, it is essential not to force them to do so. Time is a great healer and children will join in, as and when they gain overall confidence. Simple exercise can be achieved by daily walking.

When you feel ready to give exercise a go, as a safety measure, ask a Stoma Nurse or GP to examine your wounds to check that they are completely healed before attempting any sport related activity. Confirm with them when you are able to begin exercise and discuss the type of sport or exercise you have planned. Then, once you feel fit enough, begin a gradual return to sport.

As you have not used your muscles for some time, a few normal muscle aches are to be expected. Initially, you will not be at your competitive best. Slowly build up your strength and stamina before you plan the next marathon! Stop immediately if you feel any sudden or intense pain.

There are some sports to approach with caution: karate, kickboxing, and weight lifting or rough contact sports like rugby; but do not let it stop you altogether. Again, consult with your GP before you begin and follow their recommendations closely. You can wear a belt and a hard stoma cap to ensure damage limitation. Participation too soon after surgery, or without the right protection, may incur a prolapsed stoma or a hernia that would mean discomfort, pain or even further surgery.

Ostomists, particularly Ileostomists and Urostomists are more susceptible to becoming dehydrated than normal when they are active (playing sport, exercising or doing any kind of manual work), so care should be taken to drink plenty of fluid. A sign of being well hydrated is the production of 2.5 pints (four bladder's full) of urine each day. When exercising, less urine is produced making it more concentrated. It is important that you drink more to rehydrate the body. An isotonic, electrolyte or glucose drink is the recommended fluid. (See Chapter 11 for an electrolyte mix).

If you would like to discuss any concerns you may have with a fellow sports ostomate in a particular sport or in your geographical area, the Colostomy Association, Ileostomy Association or Urostomy Association will put you in touch with other players or contacts with sports associations:

www.colostomyassociation.org.uk
www.the-ia.org.uk
www.uagbi.org .uk

Once you brave the court, field, pool or gym you may not be on top form, or play as well as you used to before your operation. You may find that your reactions have slowed, perhaps because you may be overly conscious of your stoma and afraid of potential injury. However, it will only be a matter of time before you begin to take your stoma for granted and are up to speed. During contact sports, it is however only sensible to use a stoma cap to prevent accidental bumps and falls.

While you may be able to compete on an even playing field with your fellow sports people, you may find that you have difficulty with various aspects of a sport including the need for some extra facilities for dressing/changing/showering. You will need a separate toilet that includes a sink and disposal bin. Many sports centres do have disabled toilets that you can utilise to change, returning to the locker room when you are comfortably dressed.

To be sure that these facilities are available to you, the Federation of Disability Sport is a great contact point to start further investigation. It brings together people from across the country involved and interested in the development of all aspects of disability problems associated with sport:

- In England the contact is:
  www.efds.co.uk

- For Wales contact:
  www.disability-sport-wales.org

- For Scotland contact:
  www.scottishdisabilitysport.com

- For Northern Ireland contact:
  www.dsni.co.uk

These associations also provide special fitness suites all over the UK that are supervised by trained, medically qualified staff who can advise you on which machines and specific exercises are better suited to an ostomist.

Gym Activities

Visit **www.inclusivefitness.org/index.php**
to find your local fitness centre. These fitness centres provide a safe environment with special changing, toilet and shower facilities much better suited to the ostomist than some larger sports centres that lack privacy in most changing areas.

Technically all sports facilities that are open to the public should include a disabled toilet and shower. If these facilities are not available contact your regional disability sports organisation, listed above, and they will investigate further on your behalf.

It is essential that you ask the equipment supervisor as to which equipment you should or not use. If they are not familiar with an ostomate's restrictions then ask them to find out. Do not use any gym equipment until you are satisfied that is suitable for an ostomate to use. Some machines will put undue pressure on the stoma. At the very least, this may result in a burst bag or at the worst, a hernia!

Infrared saunas are perfect for an ostomate but steam saunas can result in air expansion within the bag or weakening of the bag's plastic under the heat.

Infrared saunas are also now available for in-home use as low as £400 each. They require only standard electricity and can be used only as required, taking thirty minutes to heat up to the recommended 38°C. The cabin is the size of a double wardrobe and can fit into a large bathroom or bedroom.

Contact sports/team games

For all sports other than swimming, wear a protective band. An excellent product is the **Bullen Care Fix Stoma Safe** band. This is a soft, lightweight, stretch band (in white), that will keep the stoma firmly in place. The **Bullen** belt is available on prescription. It comes in small, medium and large sizes. The size descriptions are a little misleading. The small size is suitable for schoolchildren from eight years. The medium is suitable for ladies' 10-16 sizes, men's 32-36 and the large for ladies' 18-20 sizes, men's 38-40.

Another good alternative is a maternity or "Belly band", available from Marks and Spencer, Mothercare, other maternity shops and on ebay. These come in a variety of colours and exact sizes and are extremely comfortable, disguising the stoma and its bag under sports clothing.

To find out if a firmer support belt would be useful to you, contact the Stoma Nurse to measure you accurately. An Oakmed girdle or support belt works very well for contact sports such a football or rugby.

Wear a cotton bag cover to help prevent any chaffing of the skin. (Bullen supplies these in a waterproof version for swimming or after sports showering, as well as cotton).

If your flange or pouch fits too tightly around the stoma and you do a lot of running there is a chance that the stoma will swell a little and look rather angry. This usually vanishes after a few weeks. If it does not, ask the Stoma Nurse to check it for you. A hard stoma cap is available from White Rose Collection Ltd. Excellent, if you anticipate being hit by a ball, racquet or another player!

www.bullens.com – lightweight girdles (prescription); bag covers (prescription).
www.oakmed.co.uk – firm girdle & support belt (prescription).
www.whiterosecollection.com- hard stoma cap (paid item).

Swimming

Firstly, you may be worried about the possibility of the bag or flange dropping off in the water. Be assured that most modern adhesives are designed to stay on in water, in fact the water strengthens the adhesives to make sure the bag is super secure during a swim or bathing.

Unwanted Baggage

There are special swimming costumes available from several ostomy manufacturers. These come in a variety of styles, including two-piece costumes. All these costumes are designed to both hide the bag and to ensure that it is safely held in place. Male swimmers may also prefer to wear a t-shirt/vest above their swimming trunks to hide high stoma /bag/scars.

A cheaper alternative for the ladies, is to purchase a swim dress, in a size larger than you would normally wear, to allow for generous stoma coverage. A conventional tankini is not always suitable as the tops are designed to cling and do not seem to extend beneath the bottom half. However, you can buy separates that will allow you to buy a larger size top to cover the bag. Marks and Spencer have a good range of tankini tops from as little as £7.00 and these are even cheaper during their sales.

Ostomy Specialised Swimming Costume suppliers include:
www.whiterosecollection.com
www.vblush.com
www.cuiwear.com

Swim dresses and tankinis
www.marksandspencer.com

If you wish to use your normal pouch, you can always roll the end up and tape this to your skin, the bag then becomes less obtrusive.

Another solution is to use the very small temporary bags such as the **Pelican Afresh closed Mini,** that is available in both clear and opaque or the **Dansac 229**. Pelican also manufacture a **drainable Afresh mini**. Both the Dansac and Pelican minis can be pre-cut to exact stoma sizes. Both of these are wonderful for swimming, bathing or showering but can only be worn for short periods due to the limited amount of faecal matter they can contain. Extended use may lead to bursting so it is important to check these mini bags every 30 minutes to avoid embarrassment. If you are swimming in the sea, you may find yourself far from a toilet. A drainable bag can be discreetly emptied into a waste container (such as a plastic bag with seal or empty large yoghurt pot). You can usually manage this discreetly under a towel or bathrobe/wrap.

Mini bag suppliers:
www.pelicanhealthcare.co.uk
www.dansac.co.uk

Whichever bag you wear, remember to cover it with one of the special filter covers supplied with the bags. A small amount of leakage can occur through an uncovered filter.

Riding

Riding is very possible, but may result in some strain, increased wind and also cause the bag to fill faster than normal. This is from the so-called "bounce-affect", or constant jarring on the stoma. The use of a Western saddle or specialised disabled riding saddle may reduce this quite dramatically. The organisation, **Riding for Disabled People,** provides disabled people with the opportunity to ride or carriage-drive, including the use of specialised padded saddles, and includes opportunities to join in social activities, competitions, or to take a riding holiday. Financial assistance is also available. For more information contact:

www.riding-for-disabled.org.uk

Sailing and other water sports

Sailing is a wonderful pursuit but often the mercy of the tides may leave a vessel becalmed at sea for several hours. The Royal Yacht Association's "Sailability" division aims to take the "dis", out of disability by utilising a range of sailing vessels and offering challenging pursuits for all classifications of disabled sports people – primarily it recognises that there is a continence factor to be met and ensures facilities are provided for. For more information, contact: **www.rya.org.uk**
(Search for sailability under the 'programme' tag.)

The Jubilee Sailing Trust

In addition to the RYA, the Jubilee Sailing Trust (also known as the JST) **www.jst.org.uk** is a registered charity that owns and operates *Lord Nelson* and *Tenacious*; the only two tall ships in the world to be designed and built with the purpose of enabling people of all physical abilities to sail side-by-side on equal terms. Its aims are to promote the integration of able and disabled people through the medium of tall ship sailing. Special toilets were installed, especially for ostomate sailors.

On a voyage with the Jubilee Sailing Trust, you can learn the historic art of sailing a tall ship and be involved in almost every activity on board including taking the helm, setting sails and keeping watch, regardless of your physical ability. You will discover amazing places, make great friendships and share in the challenge and adventure of sailing a tall ship on the open sea. It is why many people find a voyage with the Jubilee Sailing Trust a truly life-changing experience.

Whether you want to dip your toe in the water with a one-day *"taster"* sailing experience; spend seven days island hopping in the Canary Islands; or be part of the crew in the Tall Ships Races, the Jubilee Sailing Trust can offer you a very special experience.

Wheelyboat Trust

The Wheelyboat Trust is a registered charity dedicated to providing disabled people with the opportunity and freedom to enjoy waters large and small all over the UK. Its role is to help and encourage venues open to the public to acquire Wheelyboats (all manner of motor boats, rowboats, yachts etc.) for their disabled visitors and to help groups and organisations acquire Wheelyboats for their own use.

Wheelyboat locations are throughout the UK. The website has details of locations and the different facilities at each site.:
www.wheelyboats.org

Snow Sports

Ski suits are usually one-piece garments that are difficult put on and take off. Salopettes are a nightmare! Bending to fit skis and ski boots require a modicum of flexibility that may be beyond the average ostomate. In the UK, at Disability Snowsport, all these things are taken into consideration, especially for newcomers to the snow scene. It is a great organisation and even has temporary toilet facilities "en piste", for both skiers and snowboarders. For further information, contact:

Disability Snowsports UK
Cairngorm Mountain,
Aviemore,
PH22 1RB
01479 861272
www.disabilitysnowsport.org.uk

DSUK is a people-centred organisation with a unique sense of purpose - that anyone, regardless of his or her disability, can take part in and enjoy the thrill of snow sports.

For nearly 30 years, they have enabled those with a disability to experience the joy of skiing and snowboarding. They provide exciting and life enhancing activities for individuals or groups who require adaptive equipment and/or special instruction and support. More importantly, accessible toilets are in close proximity to the designated tutorial areas. They offer:

- Highly qualified and experienced instructional staff

- The latest developments in adaptive skiing and equipment

- Overseas activity weeks, adaptive snow sport school in Scotland, local groups, schools and youth programmes, support for the British Disabled Ski Team

- Training for instructors, volunteers and ski centre staff

- Advice and encouragement

Snow Sport's Overseas Locations
Ski 2 Freedom Foundation
www.ski2freedom.com
Email **info@ski2freedom.com**
UK: 44 (0)7980 691372
France: 33 (0)648526402
Switzerland: 41 (0)76 466 1417

This is an independent non-profit organisation created in 2007, which has established itself as a major portal to encourage snow-sport activities for those with physical difficulties, chronic long-term illnesses, carers, post-operative patients, sufferers of chronic depression and many other special needs.

Ski 2 Freedom encourages as many people as possible, regardless of age, nationality or background, to experience the exhilaration, joy, challenges and freedom of the mountains. The website offers all kinds of information to help with any assistance that their illness or condition requires. Ski 2 is based in Austria, France, Germany, Scandinavia and Switzerland.

Adventure Activities

Breakaway are the UK's only weekend activity breaks designed for young people from 4-18 with bowel and/or bladder dysfunctions and their families.Weekends are devised and organised by people with a full knowledge of living with a bowel or bladder illness.

Breakaway weekends and events offer a unique opportunity for families and young people in similar situations to meet, talk about and share their experiences, take part in confidence building action adventure activities in a relaxed and friendly environment. To find out more information about events visit:
www.breakaway-visit.co.uk

Chapter Thirteen
Travelling with a stoma
...Hints and Tips for UK and International Adventures

Before Setting Off (UK)

If you are planning to make even the shortest journey, you need to know that the whole journey can be accomplished to suit any accessible needs (including toilets). So that you can really enjoy your trip, consult the blue badge map for details of amenities and any interesting attractions en route. The website is:

bluebadge.direct.govuk

Another great website with general information from ticketing to hotels is :

www.transportdirect.info

On this website, you can plan your journey (including day trips); link it to maps and mobiles, locate car parks and toilets and even check your CO_2 consumption. On this site, the latest road works, any delays to road, rail and air transport are updated hourly.

Unwanted Baggage

Travelling abroad

Necessary Documentation

Apart from your passport, you will need am **EHIC**, European Health Insurance Card for free ***emergency*** medical treatment within the EU. *Please note that an **E111 is no longer valid** and will not be accepted for payment within the EU.*

Your EHIC also includes **some** free dental treatment or treatment at a vastly reduced cost but does not cover routine GP visits or medical check-ups. You must apply for this form at least six weeks before you travel. It not only covers costs, it contains information on what to do in an emergency in each EU country.

An EHIC application form is available from main Post Offices, online at: **www.ehic.org.uk/Internet/home.do** or by telephone on the EHIC hotline: **0845 605 0707**. If your card is lost or stolen, you must report this immediately on the same telephone number. A card is valid for five years and you can apply for a new card by telephone six months before the expiry date.

If for any reason, you have to pay for emergency medical treatment within the EU, you ***may*** be entitled to a repayment. To put in a claim, it is advisable to contact the DWP as soon as possible, preferably before you return to the UK, so that you know exactly what documentation to obtain from the provider for reimbursement. Contact the Department for Work & Pensions **0191 218 1999**

(Monday to Friday 08.00-17.00). From outside the UK: **44-191 218 1999**).

Channel Islands & the Isle of Man Health Cover Warning

On April 1st 2009, the British Government ended the long-standing, reciprocal health services agreement with the Channel Islands. On April 1st 2010, the same agreement with the Isle of Man will also end. This means that as a visitor to any of the Channel Islands or the Isle of Man you would still receive free access to treatment in A&E and casualty departments. It may include some initial treatment such as bandaging of a wound, but you must now pay for any further treatment or tests. This includes emergency treatment needed after admission to the main body of a hospital, all operations and outpatient appointments. There is no cover for repatriation to the UK.

The EHIC (European Health card) **does not cover emergency health care in the Channel Islands or the Isle of Man because they are not part of the European Union.** The best advice is to take a full travel medical insurance package before you go, ensuring all conditions are met for pre-existing illnesses or long standing conditions.

Other non-EU Health coverage

Surprisingly, many non-EU countries also offer some free emergency medical and dental treatment. If you plan

Unwanted Baggage

to travel outside the EU, visit the special NHS website for details on any free medical treatment offered in the country that you intend to visit.

www.nhs.uk/countryguidance

Travel Certificate

For the ostomate traveller, an **International Travel certificate (ITC),** is also an essential piece of luggage that you should take with you. This is a certificate printed in many languages that explains that you are carrying medical supplies and that you must have them with you at all times. It explains your urgent need for a toilet and the need for privacy through customs' inspections. As current airline restrictions prohibit the carrying of any fluid or aerosols in carry on baggage, you must insure that your emergency changing pack contains sachets of cleaning/barrier creams etc. that you may normally carry in liquid format. In addition, you may no longer carry scissors in the cabin.

You can obtain an ITC through any of the ostomy associations. **It must be countersigned by your GP.** This piece of paper will help speed your journey through the Customs and Security departments of any country to which you wish to travel.

The Colostomy/Ileostomy/Urostomy Associations all issue International Travel Certificates. Contacts are as follows:

www.colostomyassociation.org.uk
www.the-ia.org.uk
www.uagbi.org

Travelling with Medication

If you are taking prescribed medication with you, it is necessary to get an additional letter from your doctor explaining what the individual medications are for and how many you need to carry with you. This must not be a general letter but must contain specifics about the drugs and dosage. The letter should also explain medical supplies (bags etc.) and the reasons for carrying scissors in your checked baggage. This is particularly important if travelling to the US, Australia, Canada, New Zealand, South Africa and the Middle East.

Within the EU, as part of a Europe-wide agreement, GPs can prescribe up to 3 months medication for overseas travel - the maximum you are allowed to take with you if leaving the country for any reason.

Some countries have set differing limits on the amount of certain drugs that you can take into that country, despite these being for personal use or with a doctor's letter. If you take listed drugs (i.e. any morphine based drug), or more than the allowed amount, you must get an import license from the Embassy of the country to which you will be travelling.

For peace of mind, get in touch with the relevant embassy in advance to check their requirements. If you are travelling to the Middle East, importation, without the

Unwanted Baggage

correct documentation, of some prescription drugs **is illegal** and you will be subject to arrest. Ignorance of the law is no excuse. (See details under customs and excise) Make sure that you have enough medication for your whole stay. Keep a list of all medication in case you lose it or need to get more during your stay.

Your doctor may also give you a pre-prepared prescription that can be filled anywhere in the UK. Overseas, local doctors can also use this. They will verify the prescription by telephoning the originating GP to confirm your details. They will then issue you a local prescription for which you will have to pay both the GP (for his time), and the dispensing pharmacist for the cost of the prescribed drugs.

Within the EU, you can show your EHIC card, although some GPs may not accept this, you can still reclaim the charges (minus prescription costs if applicable), from the NHS on your return. Outside of the EU, depending upon the terms and conditions of your travel insurance, you may be able to claim under your policy for any loss or theft of medication. If you simply failed to take enough medication with you, you will not be able to make a claim.

Medical Insurance

Regardless of possible NHS reciprocal health coverage overseas, it is always advisable to obtain travel insurance. However, many providers of travel insurance take the view that they will not provide cover for people with pre-existing medical conditions, or if they do agree, the cost is usually exorbitant.

It is **illegal** not to declare an existing medical condition on your application and, before reimbursing you, under their terms and conditions, they will contact your GP to verify that you do not have any existing medical conditions. Ignoring this requirement has resulted in refused claims simply because they did not declare their condition(s).
Unfortunately, travel insurance is not a "luxury" – it is an essential element of any trip or holiday, whether travelling in the UK or jetting off to an exotic location. Although the NHS provides adequate treatment throughout the UK, it does not cover the costs of having to stay longer in your holiday destination to receive local treatment, or in the event of hospitalization away from home, cover the costs for any family and friends that may be travelling with you to extend their stay.

Travel insurance covers unforeseen costs for travelling companions in the event of sickness preventing your return on the intended date; this includes changing or cancelling flights due to illness; extra hotel costs and transport to and from treatment centres.

A few companies offer complete medical travel insurance to travellers with pre-existing conditions at competitive prices. These include:

- **Age Concern:**

www.ageconcern.org.uk/AgeConcern/travel_insurance.asp

Unwanted Baggage

- **All Clear**:

www.allcleartravel.co.uk

- **Free Spirit**:

www.free-spirit.com

- **Worldwide**:

www.goodhealthworldwide.com

- **Direct Travel**:

www.direct-travel.co.uk/pre-existing-medical-conditions.aspx

- **The Insurance Surgery**:

www.the-insurance-surgery.co.uk

Travel Insurance for Disabled or Chronically Ill Children

Barnardo's has teamed up with travel insurance specialists, P J Hayman and Company – Free Spirit, to offer a travel insurance package available to children, young people and their families with pre existing medical conditions.

The Free Spirit policy is specifically designed to meet the needs of these families. Any surplus generated by Barnardo's from this will be re-invested in their work with children. There are reduced premiums for people without medical conditions on the same policy.

Quotes and policies can be obtained by calling Free Spirit on **0845 260 1572**, quoting BAR3666 or on:

www.barnardos.org.uk/freespirit

Medic Alert

A simple idea could save your life!

According to the Medic Alert foundation, one in three people in the UK (that is approximately 20 million people – have a medical condition that you can't spot just by looking at them (Sound familiar??).

In many serious emergencies or in the event of an accident, you may not be able to communicate your medical problems or allergies to the paramedics that may risk a dangerous outcome.

MedicAlert® is the only **non-profit** making, registered charity providing a life-saving identification system for individuals with hidden medical conditions and allergies.

MedicAlert suggest that you should wear/carry a medic alert emblem if:

- You have any type of medical condition
- You have an allergy
- You take regular medication
- You have an unusual blood group

Unwanted Baggage

In an emergency it also essential to know who your next of kin are, as it is to know your medical details. Vital information is available on the back of your MedicAlert® Emblem.
Medical and emergency personnel can then telephone the dedicated number and, by quoting your ID number, they can receive further information such as doctor's and hospital details and your current medication.

This twenty-four hour emergency telephone service is dealt with from an emergency call centre staffed with trained personnel on hand to answer all calls, including reverse charge calls, from anywhere in the world with a translation service available in over 100 languages.. All calls are logged, with full details of the caller, the nature of the call and the response given.

Membership to the MedicAlert® service - including a tailored-made Emblem - starts at just £19.95 plus the first year's Membership at £25. As a registered charity, The MedicAlert Foundation <u>can also provide free membership to individuals on a limited income</u>. Your GP may carry registration leaflets or:

To join or for further queries, call **0800 581 420 or online at <u>www.medicalert.org.uk</u>**

If illness Occurs -

If you feel unwell, run a temperature, develop a rash or any stoma related problem (diarrhoea, increase in output etc.), then <u>do not hesitate</u> to call your either your holiday representative, the hotel manager or the local pharmacy.

They will offer assistance in locating a doctor, or arranging for a clinic appointment. If in any doubt, visit the local A&E. You may need. Do not ignore symptoms, it is better to address a small problem than end up spending time in hospital instead of the beach.

Supplies to take with you

Do not presume that you can obtain bags and other ostomy supplies abroad easily. When you plan your stay, work out the number of bags you normally use and take double the amount.

Many bag manufacturers have agents abroad so before you go, ask for the name and contact address of the relevant firm in the country to which you are travelling. If there are any problems, you can contact them. If your luggage is mislaid, some UK based suppliers will provide express services to overseas patients in distress. Check with your current supplier for international contact numbers. **UK 800 numbers do not work** from international telephones.

Fittleworth provides a UK bag and supply liaison service known as the **Worldwide Assist Alliance**. This is an agreement that supports international ostomy travellers with all stoma or continence needs. By calling Fittleworth in the UK, they will arrange through their partner organisations, to deliver the necessary goods or advice and even arrange for a local stoma nurse to visit if required. **www.fittleworth.net** or by telephone: **0800 378 846**

Worldwide Assist Alliance is currently available in the following countries (although more are added on a regular basis):

- Australia
- Austria
- Belgium
- Canada
- France
- The Netherlands
- New Zealand
- Portugal
- Spain
- USA

Vaccinations

A very useful website, **www.travelturtle.co.uk**, will advise you on country specific medical and vaccination reports usually only available to registered UK healthcare professionals. It details listings of all major travel vaccines, including:

- Pertinent information in regards to the delivery method of each travel vaccine.
- Who can have the vaccine , and its compatibility with other treatments.

- Information about costs, and where it can be obtained.
- Contemporary data about who provides the service and its length of protection.

The site is new and some of the links are not yet completed but the vaccination chart is extremely good.

Water to go....

Global medical census agrees that all ostomates drink a lot more fluids than the average person must. Ostomates are also more susceptible to waterborne bacterial infections resulting in extreme diarrhoea and dehydration. It is only sensible to take precautions and although the following advice may seem a little OTT, after months of preparation and expense an enjoyable holiday ruined, simply by **H^2O!**

In hot climates, fluid intake must be increased. The most common causes of illness from drinking water in foreign countries are bacterial. However, there are still some risks of viral presence or indeed chemical pollution.

There is also the risk of illusion in that it is common for locals of a particular region to be unaffected by their tap water. Even expatriates may declare, "It is safe to drink the local water - it does not affect us!" That is because their bodies are accustomed to its impurities and have developed the appropriate immune response

Any food that has been in contact with water for the sake of rinsing, soaking or mixing can take on the same

Unwanted Baggage

risks. (e.g. salads, melon, raw vegetables etc.). If you are preparing these yourself, then use bottle water. Cooking other washed food will eliminate the bacteria.

Water is still water when it is frozen. Most impurities remain unaffected by freezing, including many bacteria. You can drink bottled water for your entire trip, but one spoonful of locally made ice cream or delicious sorbet may be a bite too far! A packaged frozen product is usually screened at source for bacteria and is a much better choice.

Cubed or crushed ice is added as standard practice to most mixed drinks, sodas and juices served abroad. One reason is that this uses less liquid, thereby saving money! Do not hesitate to ask for your drinks without potentially bacterially infected ice

The bathroom uses the same water coming from the same pipes and can inadvertently enter your mouth and even your eyes through washing. Use bottled water to clean your teeth and rinse your contact lenses. Run the shower for at least two minutes before entering the cubicle, this will ensure that any bacterium in the showerhead is flushed out. Keep your mouth closed in the shower. This may sound silly but if you start to sing, your delightful music could be inviting in those microbes.

Waterborne bacteria can also enter through the stoma, so ensure that you keep your bag on at all times in the shower or bath. Use only boiled or bottled water or a stoma cleansing solution to clean the stoma.

An antibacterial hand gel is a good, safe method of washing hands. This is available, on prescription, for ostomates in individual sachet or pump container format (Ostagel).

In the UK and overseas, more and more hotels and local authorities are turning to alternate, environmentally friendly methods of maintaining the Ph balance in swimming pools, thereby avoiding the use of chlorine. Some of these methods, while keeping the pool "sparkling", may not necessarily kill waterborne bacteria. This in turn, has caused a marked increase in bacterial infections through swallowing pool water. While enjoying a good swim, be careful to keep your mouth closed and avoid anything that may cause inadvertent ingestion of pool water.

How to combat dehydration:

- Bottled water is the safest and most commonly advised prescription. Find out the name of a reliable, local brand and ensure that the cap is sealed. One hotel in a very exclusive resort in southern Spain was fined for refilling bottles with tap water!

- Boiling is the best way to sterilize water. Tea and coffee are therefore safe options. Boiling water, and allowing it to cool before drinking, is the most efficient and inexpensive sterilisation method. Remember to keep the water covered while it cools. Travel kettles can be purchased, with the relevant electrical adaptors, at most airport/ferry retail outlets.

- As with imported frozen foods, canned and sealed bottled drinks are generally safe. If you can trust the name, then you can trust the contents.

- Have a beer! Alcohol kills the yeast used to make it and any bacterial content; hence, alcoholic beverages are usually clean. When choosing a mixer however, ask for a can or bottled soda or juice as an accompaniment. The on-tap variety is made from a mix with local water added.

- In addition, you should know that a large intake of caffeine or alcohol increases the effects of dehydration.

If you fall ill, stay hydrated. If the symptoms become severe or it do not clear up within two days, you must consult a local physician, explaining that you are an ostomate. You may also wish to take extra loperamide for an immediate solution but this should not replace advice from a doctor or pharmacist.

Food

The most common travel related illnesses are gastrointestinal infections that can be dangerous to ostomates. These infections are mainly due to untreated water but also poorly prepared food, a common occurrence in all countries.

If you experience the following, visit a medical professional immediately:

- High Fever (greater than 38.9°C/102°F)
- Shaking chills
- Severe Headaches
- Stiff neck
- Unusual Abdominal pain
- Unusual Muscle and Joint pain
- Pronounced skin rash
- Yellow skin/eyes
- Continual fluid output into the bag (ostomates)
- Diarrhoea/strong colour urine (urostomates)

Foods that may be unsafe include:

- Food from street vendors
- Shellfish
- Unpasteurised milk/dairy products
- Thin skinned fruit such as grapes
- Salads, such as lettuce
- Food unprotected from flies

Cover your bag in the sun

If you like spending lots of time in the sun, it is best to cover your bag with a cotton bag cover. These are available on prescription and help to stop your skin sweating under the plastic of the bag. This in turn, prevents any infection or rash near the stoma.

Accidents

Leakage from bags and occasional bursting of bags happens. Always carry your emergency kit in your carry-on baggage. Aircraft pressure can build up inside the bag and, if left unchecked, can cause bursting. You should pop to the toilet every 30 minutes in flight to keep an eye on the bag. On long haul flights if you check the bag for the first two hours and are happy that no excess wind has built up, then you should be able to sleep for a few hours without worrying.

Carry a change of clothes in carry-on luggage in case the worst happens. Make sure that the on board toilet has plenty of toilet paper and hand towels prior to using. If you have an emergency and, by chance, all the toilets are occupied ask the flight attendants who will either send you to a toilet in another flight class or allow you to use the staff toilet (yes, there is one on all the larger planes!).

If you are travelling on a smaller, single class plane then the flight attendants may knock at the toilet doors to ask the occupant to hurry up. Many people use the toilet for private space to apply make up etc. and no-one minds being disturbed in an emergency. It is much better to ask than to become anxious about problems.

You can also advise the cabin staff on boarding or at the check-in counter that you are wearing a bag and this will alert them to the possibility that bags are subject to air pressure (on which they will have been trained), and will be only too happy to help if there are any problems..

If you are worried about embarrassing accidents whilst staying in a hotel, take a few disposable bed mats, (available on prescription from **Bullens Healthcare**), so that the mattress will not be damaged. If an accident happens then ask the hotel management to change the bedding immediately.

All manner of accidents happen and hotels are used to it. You must not spoil your holiday by blaming yourself over a situation you cannot control. If you feel uncomfortable, ask the management to leave a spare set of bedding in the room.

Customs and excise

Travelling with Medication and medical supplies

Due to restrictions on many flights across the globe, those travelling with existing medical conditions need to be aware of restrictions when travelling with medication. Some airlines now restrict the amount of hand luggage allowed on flights, it is essential to check with your individual airline prior to flying. Many airlines restrict the amount of fluid medications and may insist on these carried in clear plastic bags. Regulations are changing all the time. It is essential that you check with your specific airline the day before departure.

The Chief Medical Officer in the UK has issued a procedure for those taking medication on flights (Department of Health 2006).

- It states that travellers should be discouraged from taking medication onto flights unless it is for the immediate journey and an allowance of time at the other end to pick up your baggage (allow at least 4 hours).

- It also recommends that all extra supplies of medication for your arrival be placed in the hold luggage.

- Any powder/inhalers or tablets can be carried in the hand luggage - up to 50 grams.

- Any liquids, creams or gel medications, that are essential for the flight, may be carried in hand luggage as long as they are smaller than 50ml (such as a GTN spray).

- If the amount is larger than 50mls, you might be asked to taste it – the airports have plastic cups available for this procedure!

- If an adult is travelling with a young child and wants to carry non-prescription medication onto the flight they will need to taste the child's medication (as long as they are not allergic to it!).

- All medication involving syringes must be carried with sealed syringes. Carrying Syringes by themselves is not allowed, even if they are sealed.

- Whilst on board, Airline staff may retain your medication in a locked cabinet. This is at the discretion of the airline/pilot.

The DOH issues these regulations and any updates are on the DOH website.

Benefit letters

You should carry proof of disability. (All ostomy patients are entitled to Disability Living Allowance). You should carry proof of DLA or incapacity allowance if applicable. This verifies your entitlement to assistance, extra baggage allowances and the benefit of a private security search. If you are not claiming benefits, you may carry a letter from your GP instead. This should briefly outline your condition, explaining your need for privacy searches and for an extra baggage allowance for your ostomy supplies.

Every country has different provisions for those needing accessible toilets. Be prepared for the worst. If you are in any doubt about international travel accessibility (i.e. foreign airport toilets etc.), ask your travel agent to check for you and put into writing the kind of facilities you can expect at your destination. If you ask them to put the information in writing, they are more likely to carry out a thorough search on your behalf rather than a guesstimate. Recently, a friend arrived at an obscure airport and found that even the airport toilets little more than holes in the ground; not the "perfectly good accessible toilets" they were told about. It was lucky that they carried a disposable "*Traveljohn*" into which they were able to empty their bag. These useful items are available from:
www.whiterosecollection.com

www.cleanseatuk.com

Air Travel

Since July 26th 2008, new EU regulations have been introduced to give disabled air travellers improved airport access rights. Under the new law, you do **not** need to be in a wheelchair, permanently ill or physically disabled to enjoy these enhanced rights.

Anyone who has a disability, chronic illness or temporary condition can benefit from these extra facilities and assistance.

Discounted airport parking

For details of discounted airport parking for blue badge holders or those in receipt of Disability Living Allowance or Incapacity benefit, check :

www.helpmetravel.co.uk

Airport Car Parks

These car parks have to provide additional spaces for blue badge holders and "Help points" where assistance must be available to get disabled passengers through the entire process to board their flights.

Disabled passengers must be the first to board aircraft and after disembarking, airport staff must help them retrieve their baggage. Queries by telephone are on these general numbers:

- **0845 604 6610 England**
- **0845 604 8810 Wales**
- **0845 604 5510 Scotland**

Airport and Airline Security

The safety and security of passengers is a priority. All passengers must pass through security control before they enter the departure lounges. Wheelchair users will inevitably activate the archway metal detector, and security personnel are obliged to hand-search passengers who activate alarms; therefore, chair and passenger will be searched.

As you are wearing an ostomy bag, you can ask to be searched in private, away from the main security control area. Do not be embarrassed to request this, it an important right and necessary to maintain your dignity in these situations.

Luggage

It is a good idea to carry some bags and cleansing supplies in a carry-on case as well as in your checked luggage – that way if something goes missing, you will have a back up until you can obtain more supplies.

Mobility Aids

In addition to your standard baggage allowance, aircraft will also carry one lightweight, foldable, manual wheelchair per passenger free of charge in the aircraft hold. However, for mobility aids in excess of 32kgs, special permission must be requested when bookings are made because of weight and space restrictions.

Evidence must also be provided at check-in that the passenger is registered disabled. If the above criteria are not met, the mobility aid will be charged as excess baggage by its weight.

Aircraft seating

In the economy section on all aircraft, several seats at the front of the section are normally held for passengers with reduced mobility or for those who may have an urgent need to access the toilet (and their companions). These seats are close to the front entrance and the onboard WC facilities.

You should notify the airline's customer service department in writing or email and keep a copy of the acknowledgement. Explain your needs and ask what your rights are to guaranteed seating.

If you check-in two hours prior to departure and you have a confirmed mobility assistance place, you will be guaranteed a seat at the front of your section, and the check-in staff will make every effort to seat you before other passengers embark.

Mandatory Airline forms

If you have a, long-term disability or stable medical condition, or fly regularly with one airline, the carrier may not require you to complete these forms. If you are unsure, check with your airline before purchasing your ticket.

However, if you have any medical needs, the airline *may* ask you to complete an Incapacitated Passengers Handling Advice **(INCAD)** form and/or a Medical Information Form **(MEDIF).**

Issued by all airlines, these standard forms help staff organise any assistance/equipment you may need during your journey. With some airlines, the INCAD and MEDIF are two parts of the same form.

You can fill in the INCAD form yourself; your doctor must complete the MEDIF form, in advance. Do check with each individual carrier well in advance of your flight, as this paperwork must be completed beforehand saving disappointment and possible cancellation of your flight.

The MEDIF and INCAD forms are only applicable for one journey. If you are a frequent air traveller, you can get a Frequent Traveller Medical Card (FREMEC).

This is available from most airlines and gives the airline a permanent record of your specific needs. This means you will not have to fill in a form and make special arrangements every time you fly. However, if you change airlines (from the one that originally issued your FREMEC

Unwanted Baggage

card), you should check that the alternate airline will also accept it.

Airport Accessibility information

For any general airport information, please check :
www.ukairportguide.co.uk

For the main UK airports, accessibility information is as follows:

Heathrow Airport
www.heathrowairport.com

BAA Heathrow has responsibility for providing assistance at the airport and the airlines assume this responsibility when you are on board the aircraft. If you have a disability, chronic illness or you experience mobility problems and need assistance on arrival at the airport, or with boarding, you must inform your airline **and** the airport of your particular need at least forty-eight hours before you fly.

It is advisable to give as much notice as possible for both the outbound and return journey, this way they can ensure you receive the assistance you require. If, however, no notification is made, the airport will still make all reasonable efforts to assist you.

- Even if you are mobile, there can be long distances within the airports themselves and any assistance (by means of en electric trolley), might be useful.

- A long wait, standing at a check in counter, unable to leave your luggage to make a very necessary toilet trip can make your whole journey miserable and embarrassing. It is better to ask for help beforehand rather than try to find assistance in a busy airport.

- As well as informing the airline, you may wish to inform the special assistance provider at Heathrow Airport (contact details below).

- To receive assistance you must arrive at a designated point no later than two hours before the published flight departure time, or you must present yourself for check-in no later than one hour before the published departure time.

- All registered disabled passengers are entitled to use the VIP check in desks.

- Help points are located on terminal forecourts, short-stay car parks, in stations and in baggage reclaim halls.

Heathrow Special Assistance Provider's Contact details:

Terminal 1,	02087452165
Terminal 2,	020 8745 2195
Terminal 3	020 8745 2227
Terminal 4,	020 8745 2357
Terminal 5,	020 3165 0285

Reserved seating areas

Reserved seating areas are available for disabled passengers. These are identified by the use of special needs pictograms, and are located in all terminals within the general seating areas. They aim to have the following features:

- Low-level flight information screens.
- Arms on both sides of seats.
- Space for wheelchair users.

Toilets

Appearances are deceptive, many ostomates' physical appearance conceals their actual needs and some people may question your use of the accessible toilets. You have more pressing needs than concerns with other peoples' opinions – Ignore them – you do not have to explain yourself. If questioned by an official of the airport, simply show them your "toilet needs card", available from CROHN'S AND COLITIS UK, the colostomy, ileostomy or urostomy associations.

Most toilet blocks include a unisex accessible toilet nearby. Occasionally an individually accessible toilet is located inside the men's' and ladies' toilets. Please note that abled parents travelling with children of the opposite sex may also use the accessible toilets.

Airport Shopping

If you want to do some pre-flight duty-free shopping but hate struggling with the extra bags, you can use airport "Shop & Collect" whereby your purchases will be delivered to your aircraft.

"Shop & Collect" is a FREE service, available when you are flying within the EU (including flights within the UK). If you are purchasing duty free goods for your return, Shop &Collect will also store your goods securely whilst you are away and insure them. Upon your return to the airport, they will be ready and waiting for you at a convenient collection point, after you have claimed your luggage and cleared customs.

To use the service, simply tell the assistant in-store that you would like to "Shop & Collect", show your boarding card details and they will take care of the rest for you. This convenient service means you can shop in all stores and still not have to carry anything. This service also lets you take advantage of time-limited special offers. In addition, it is a great way to get around the current restrictions on carrying liquids on your return flight.

Gatwick Airport
www.gatwickairport.com
The details for check in, security, seating, shopping and toilets are the same as for Heathrow although some arrangements have recently changed. BAA Gatwick now has responsibility at the airport and the airlines are responsible when you are on board the aircraft.

As well as informing the airline, you may wish to inform G4S, the special assistance provider at Gatwick is: **01293 507 502**

Stanstead Airport
www.stansteadairport.com
The details for check in, security, seating, shopping and toilets are the same as for Heathrow.
You can contact the special assistance provider at Stanstead Airport is: **07715 171 316**

Glasgow Airport
www.glasgowairport.com
The details for check in, security, seating and toilets are the same as for Heathrow.
The special assistance provider is on 0141 842 7700 at Glasgow Airport. Email: **info@thsscotland.co.uk**

Edinburgh Airport
www.edinburghairport.com
The details for check in, security, seating and toilets are the same as for Heathrow.
The special assistance provider at Edinburgh Airport is on: **0131 344 3449**

Aberdeen Airport
www.aberdeenairport.com
The details for check in, security, seating, shopping and toilets are the same as for Heathrow.
The special assistance provider at Aberdeen Airport is on; **01224 725767.**

Elizabeth Prosser & Philip Prosser

Manchester Airport
www.manchesterairport.co.uk

If you have not pre-arranged assistance, passengers requiring assistance into Manchester Airport are able to contact the service provider OCS by using the designated blue courtesy phones provided. These are located by the entrance doors to the Terminal Buildings, and the Bus and Rail Station.

OCS will collect you and will assist you to the check-in desk. There is no shopping assistance at Manchester Airport. Due to recent security problems, **drop off and collection at the departure/arrivals terminal is no longer possible**. You can contact the airport to arrange pick-up from the car parks.

To pre-arrange assistance, telephone Manchester Airport Customer Service on: **0871 271 0711**

A Reception Point for Assistance is also available in the check-in hall of each Terminal. OCS is present to greet passengers and to coordinate assistance from this point to the departure gate.

Accessible areas include enhanced seating, which is higher than standard seating and has retractable armrests to help passengers transfer in and out of their seat and low flight information monitors.

Terminal 1 – is located opposite check in desk 22
Terminal 2 – is located opposite check in desk 50
Terminal 3 – is located opposite check in desk 37

Unwanted Baggage

Passengers may choose to remain in their own wheelchair or may choose to one provided by OCS.

OCS has a range of specialist equipment to help you board your aircraft efficiently and will discuss your individual requirements and arrange the most appropriate type of help.

Your return journey

OCS staff will assist passengers from the aircraft, through Immigration to the Baggage Reclaim Hall.

Once you have collected your baggage, OCS will assist you to your final point of onward travel such as Car park, Bus and Rail Station.

Cardiff Airport
info.cwlfly.com/en

Cardiff International Airport assists passengers with mobility problems arriving at the airport. The following facilities are available at three special assistance call points located in the car parks and outside the main entrance of the outbound terminal. Special assistance passengers can be helped from check in, through to security, into the departure lounge and onto the aircraft.

Inbound special assistance passengers can be assisted to disembark the aircraft and taken through passport control, customs and the baggage hall. Passengers can also be assisted back to the special assistance points in the car parks or to the public transport facilities available.

Passengers are advised to pre-book with their tour operator or airline or directly with Cardiff International

Airport by contacting: **01446 729329** or e-mailing: **PRMDesk@cwl.aero**

Additional facilities include:
- Dedicated spaces in the car parks
- Low level kerbs at terminal entrance and exit
- Use of airport wheelchairs throughout terminal building
- Passengers may retain their own wheelchairs up until boarding - please check with your airline
- Lifts between all floors
- Specially designated toilets on the first floor, departure lounge and arrivals hall
- A special assistance waiting area in the departure lounge is available with low level courtesy phone and flight information
- Fast-track for wheelchair and special assistance passengers at security central search
- Ambulift for boarding aircraft

Bristol Airport
www.bristolairport.co.uk
For all passengers who require assistance, contact OCS help desk on: **01275 473403**.

Unwanted Baggage

Bristol Airport facilities include:

- Lifts to all floors.
- Wheelchairs and a help desk for passengers with accessibility problems.
- The disabled toilets all have help buttons.
- No shopping assistance is provided.

The Car Park facilities include:

- Help buttons on entry barriers and payment machines.
- Larger bays in the long and short term car parks
- Wheelchair-friendly minibuses for transfer to the terminal building.

PLEASE NOTE: Due to terrorism concerns, pick up and drop off is not permitted on the Terminal Forecourt.

Customers requiring assistance should go to the Pick up/Drop off Car Park, located adjacent to the terminal building. Help can be requested through the intercom system at the payment machine or the entry barrier.

Birmingham Airport
www.bhx.co.uk

Blue Badge drivers and passengers can enjoy a thirty-minute complimentary parking facility in the Rapid Drop-Off area. To obtain the free parking, drivers should go to the NCP Customer Service Desk in the Link Building between the two terminals prior to leaving the Airport and show their Blue Badge to get their car park ticket validated.

Passengers requiring special assistance should call OCS on 0121 767 7878, who will assess individual circumstances and arrange help through the airport terminal to your aircraft.

If you require wheelchair assistance to the terminal from the car parks; from the check-in desks to the aircraft; or on arriving back at Birmingham International Airport; OCS staff will escort you from the aircraft, through immigration & customs and assist you in retrieving your luggage. To arrange this please contact your tour operator or airline in the first instance. If you need to contact OCS directly, the helpdesk number is:**0121 767 7878.** The Special Assistance Reception Desk is located on the Ground Floor of Terminal Two. Help points are located within this area linked to the OCS helpdesk.

Airport Layout Maps

The Directgov Blue Badge map website has airport plans for twenty UK airports. The plans show the layout of the airport and the location of various facilities. This includes check-in desks, car parking, accessible toilets, information desks and more.

www.bluebadge.direct.gov.uk/index.php?br_wid=1024&br_hgt=768

Unwanted Baggage

International airport information is available from the countries' embassies or by web search for the relevant airports.

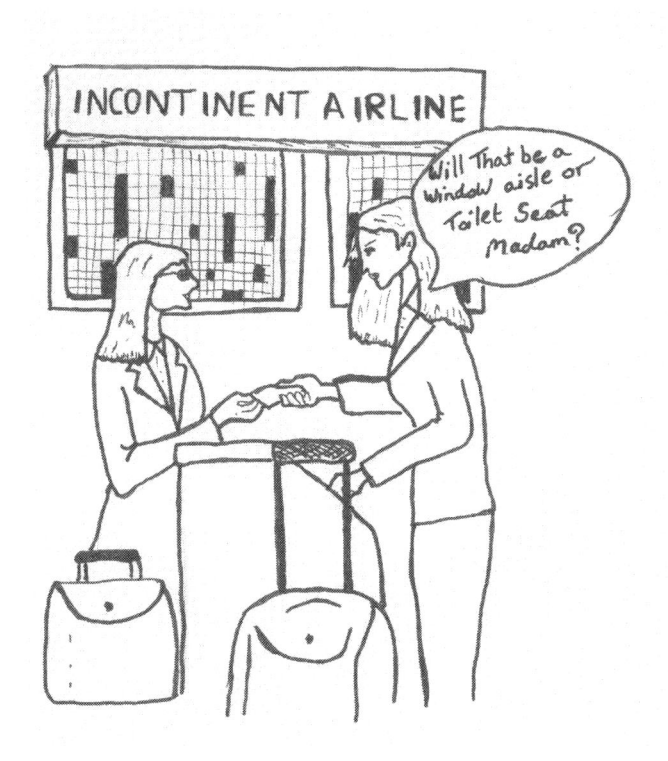

Airport Check-In

You must check-in two hours before the scheduled flight time so that you receive the pre-booked assistance and to ensure that you are taken to the aircraft in plenty of time. If you do not need mobility assistance, but can book an airline seat in advance, make sure you book an aisle set, preferably near the toilet. Explain to the airline that you will have to visit the toilet unexpectedly, as the air pressure can cause the bag to expand and the excess air will need releasing to prevent bursting. Check with your travel agent or airline who, even if pre-booking is not standard, they may be willing to make exceptions for your medical condition.

Security Checks

There are different types of security checks at different airports. Be ready to explain the medical equipment that you are carrying in your hand luggage. If the security team needs to do a more thorough search, then security staff should:

- Ensure each stage of the process is explained in clear and simple words.

- Offer the option of a private area to perform the search.

- Listen to what you have to say and consider your needs and act upon them as best they can.

- Offer help at any stage of the search if you need it.

- Offer a blanket or similar during a search.

- Security staff should handle any medication discreetly and re-pack it carefully.

Unwanted Baggage

In Transit

Make sure you have your pocket travel kit with your quick-change items to hand. You may also wish to carry a change of clothing and underpants for any emergency. If you have not been able to pre-book a seat, plan to arrive early to ensure an aisle seat at least. Once on the plane and in the air you can expect the bag to balloon a little due to the change in cabin pressure. If left unattended, it may burst! Make frequent trips to the toilet to ensure the release of trapped air. Avoid any fizzy drinks, as this will make the ballooning worse.

Do not hesitate to make the aircraft staff aware of your situation and make sure you call them from the toilet if you need any help.

You may wish to order a special meal if you are on any dietary restrictions. This must be pre-arranged with the carrier either through your travel agent or directly with the carrier.

Once on the ground, your stoma content output may be liquid for a few days, but will soon settle down again into its usual pattern.

Train Travel

If you have difficulty with mobility or have a chronic illness, special arrangements can be made for disabled passengers. If you are in receipt of Disability Living Allowance or Incapacity Benefit, you are entitled to a disabled Persons Railcard. National Rail will also issue this card on production of a GP letter explaining your need for assistance. Application details can be found at: **www.disabledpersons-railcard.co.uk**

This card entitles you, <u>and an accompanying passenger,</u> to one third off rail fares. More importantly, it allows you access to the disabled lounges and their excellent toilet facilities, present on all major UK stations. These lounges provide special ticketing booths to assist you with any problems you have in transit.

The Railcard also offers a number of discounts and offers including:

- Twenty percent off meals/snacks at designated outlets on or near 120 UK stations. You can apply online at:

  www.bitecard.co.uk/register.asp?mode=doit

- Over 100 "two for one" offers at top London attractions, restaurants, theatres and much more. Combine your visit with Free London activities and see lots more suggestions in the London Culture Guide. **www.daysoutguide.co.uk**

- The booklet "**Rail Travel Made Easy**" provides useful information for disabled passengers.

Maps for People with "**Reduced Mobility**

Maps" showing which stations have access to platforms without the use of steps and accessible toilet locations

Unwanted Baggage

- If you are a parent of a child in receipt of Disability Living Allowance, a children's fare already offers a fifty percent discount. However, if you obtain a Disabled Person's Railcard, this enables the accompanying adult to travel at the reduced rate of one third off.

Once you have your card, your can arrange for railway staff to meet you at your departure station, accompany you to the train and see you safely on board. Similar arrangements can be made at your destination station and other stations if you need to change trains. An electric trolley will be made available at all major rail stations to take you to taxi ranks, toilets etc.

To see which Train Operating Company you need to contact for assistance and to find out about station facilities, check the railcard website.

London Residents:

If you are a London resident and over 60 or in receipt of Disability Living Allowance, you are entitled to a Freedom Pass which offers free travel on all of London's public transport network.
www.tfl.gov.uk/tickets/faresandtickets/1065.aspx

EUROPEAN TRAIN TRAVEL
Some journeys and train companies across Europe offer special discounted passes for travellers in receipt of Disability Living Allowance and may allow a companion to travel with you at a reduced rate. Check what is on offer before making a booking.

Elizabeth Prosser & Philip Prosser

Mobilise

Mobilise members also qualify for a discount on Eurotunnel. See the website for details:

www.mobilise.info
For **Eurostar's** discounts and information:
www.eurostar.com/UK/uk/leisure/travel_information/ before_you_go/special_travel_needs Jsp

Travelling by Road

If you are in receipt of Disability Living Allowance, then Mobilise is your ideal road-travelling companion! The **Mobilise Organisation** was formed in 2005 from a merger of two long-standing charities, the Disabled Drivers` Association and the Disabled Drivers` Motor Club. Mobilise is *not* just an organisation for drivers, they also support passengers, scooter and wheelchair users, families and carers.

Mobilise provides information and guidance to enable people to make informed decisions about their individual transportation requirements by road and ferry. Mobilise offers good concessions on hotels, ferries, roadside rescue service and a number of other travelling aids. For more information, contact:
www.mobilise.info

It also produces information sheets and UK road maps that show parking and toilet facilities.

Unwanted Baggage

If you are travelling by road, try to plan the journey breaks around places that have adequate toilet facilities. Most roadside cafes, restaurants, service stations and hotels have accessible toilets.

www.parkingforbluebadges.com
This website provides details of the nearest toilets, blue badge parking with exact mapping and directions.

The road map, **Gowrings Mobility UK Road Atlas** details all toilets, disabled accessible beaches, city street maps with blue badge parking bays, concessions for blue badge holders, a directory of useful services, service station facilities and toll bridges. Normally selling at £12.99, it is available through *Mobilise* at a discounted rate.

On the road in the UK or abroad, you may find yourself with a long distance between facilities. If you have an emergency and need to empty a bag, **White Rose and Clean Seat UK** offers a wonderful disposable product: "Traveljohn" into which you can empty your bag discreetly.
www.whiterosecollection.com
www.cleanseatuk.com

Travelling by Bus or Coach

By Bus
For details on any bus service, contact the National Federation of Bus Users:
www.bususers.org

There are no bus services that provide on board toilets, although the local councils usually provide toilet locations in relation to bus stops.

Each local council administers different schemes for disabled bus passengers. Ask your council about their concessionary fares scheme.
The government guidelines state that concessionary (free or discounted) travel should be offered if an eligible person is someone who:

- Is blind or partially sighted.
- Is profoundly or severely deaf.
- Is without speech.
- Has a disability or chronic illness
- Has suffered an injury, which has a substantial and long-term adverse effect on his ability to walk.
- Does not have arms or has long-term loss of the use of both arms.
- Has a learning disability that would prevent them from applying for a driving licence.
- Is on medication, the effects of which would prevent them from driving.
- Otherwise, under the Road Traffic Act, an application has been refused due to the grounds of persistent misuse of drugs or alcohol.

Unwanted Baggage

By Coach

Concessionary fares

A Concessionary fare (discounted), applies to all passengers who qualify as disabled, as described by the legislation in the Transport Act 2000. This includes all recipients of DLA, Incapacity or those who can provide proof of chronic illness from their GP. The scheme applies equally to both UK residents and overseas visitors.

The concessionary fare is available on National Express services to destinations within England and Wales, and to Edinburgh or Glasgow from destinations in England and Wales. Concessionary travel is also available on summer seasonal express coach services and on Eurolines services 920 and 921 for travel to destinations within mainland Britain.

On occasion, disabled passengers may be asked to produce a local authority concessionary travel pass or other identification. Passengers should be prepared to produce this proof of eligibility at any point during their journey if requested.

Disabled passengers should always be offered a concessionary fare. If you are not offered this discount, please alert the sales person of your eligibility. For any questions, please contact the Disabled Persons Travel Helpline on: **08717 818179.**

Elizabeth Prosser & Philip Prosser

Wheelchair accessibility

National Express is introducing a new generation of coaches onto the UK network that feature a wheelchair lift incorporated into the passenger entrance.

The easy access coach features a wider entrance and a completely flat floor throughout the coach to aid mobility for all. A streamlined NX Magic Floor Lift is incorporated into the passenger entrance and when deployed, the wheelchair is locked in place and the customer safely and securely uses the same standard three-point seat belt as other customers. Other accessible features include reclining leather seats, air conditioning and a large toilet. Currently, most coaches have a standard toilet.

A programme of routes is currently being planned to roll-out the accessible coach across the network, with the whole network being fully accessible by 2012.

Routes with accessible coaches

The following services are already operating with easy access vehicles. The majority of locations along these routes can be used by the easy access coach and wheelchair users, but please contact our Disabled Persons' Travel Helpline for further information before travelling.

240 Leeds - Sheffield - Coventry - Heathrow Airport - Gatwick Airport
314 Liverpool- Stoke - Birmingham - Coventry - Northampton - Bedford – Cambridge
333 Blackpool - Bolton - Manchester - Stoke - Bristol - Yeovil - W'mouth - Poole - B'mouth
337 Coventry - Leamington - Stratford - Cheltenham - Bristol - Exeter – Torquay – Paignton

Unwanted Baggage

341 Burnley - Blackburn - Bolton - Manchester - B'ham - Weston-S-M - Exeter - Torquay (not including night or seasonal services)
390 Hull (Docks) - Leeds – Manchester
403 Bath - Swindon - Chippenham - Heathrow - London (side-entry passenger lift)
538 The Midlands - Manchester Airport - Manchester - Preston - Carlisle – Scotland
560 Barnsley - Sheffield - London (not including night or seasonal services)
562 Hull - Doncaster – London
591 Edinburgh - Newcastle - London (not including night or seasonal services)
737 Oxford - High Wycombe - Luton Airport - Stansted Airport
767 Nottingham - Leicester - Luton Airport - Stanstead Airport

Travelling By Sea

Port Facilities

There are hundreds of ports in the UK. Most offer accessible toilets and blue badge parking. In an emergency, showers are also available in the freight lounges.

Customers with any special needs are advised to contact their ferry operator prior to travelling. For detailed information about any UK port or vessel, please see the website:
www.directferries.co.uk/routes.htm

Dover

Dover is the main port of departure/entry to/ from the UK. For details of its facilities, port toilets and blue badge parking facilities, telephone: **01304 240400**

If you are a blue badge holder, you can park in the reserved parking bays in a specially designated car park. To use this car park, you will need to show your card at the Information Desk in the Travel Centre. Staff will then issue you with a windscreen disc that will permit you to enter and use this designated car park for unlimited subsequent visits.

Please note that a pay and display scheme operates at this car park, so you need to have your money available when you arrive.

Toilets

Unisex accessible toilet facilities are available in various locations throughout the Ferry Terminal.

Foot Passenger Transfers between Terminal and Ferries

Check with your ferry operator about the availability of space on the mobility bus from the Travel Centre or Embarkation Lounge. A port bus service operates from Embarkation to the ferries, and from the ferries to Arrivals.

Check with each Ferry Company, cruise operator or travel agent for detailed facilities on each individual ferry.

If you are planning to take your car and you are the driver, some ferry companies as well as Eurotunnel

Unwanted Baggage

may offer a reduction in price. See mobilise for detailed information.
www.mobilise.info

For on board toilet facilities on the following ferries contact:

P&O Ferries
Helpline: **08716 645645**
website: **www.poferries.com**
For those customers with mobility and other health issues P&O Ferries have endeavoured to provide facilities to ensure that journeys are as comfortable as possible.

- If notified or requested staff will meet and assist customers with wheelchairs on the vehicle deck. There are also wheelchairs available on board and these can be provided to the vehicle deck if requested in advance.

- There are lifts on all ships, which are wheelchair friendly.

- Disabled toilets can be found on decks 7 and 8.

- All shopping, dining and seating areas are wheelchair friendly.

Sea France
Customer support: **0871 423 7119.**
Website: **www.SeaFrance.com**
Sea France provides disabled toilets and other assistance on request. Call for information and to arrange assistance.

Stena Line
Special needs helpline: **01255 252252**
Website: **www.stenaline.co.uk**

Stena Line travellers with special needs will find a number of facilities and assistance available. There is also a disabled ferry cabin that is spacious and comes complete with its own fully accessible toilet. There is no extra charge to use this cabin beyond the standard cabin rate but this cabin must be pre-booked. In the ferry's public areas, there is a disabled toilet near the Metropolitan Restaurant on Deck 7.

Stena Line's special needs travellers will also receive assistance from a member of the onboard team in the unlikely event that there is an emergency during your ferry journey.

All other Ferry Lines

All other ferry lines are listed together with their and special needs assistance information:

Helpline: 0871 222 33121
website: **www.ferries.co.uk**

Cruising

Some cruise operators may require you to have medical clearance/certification. Check with the cruise operator or your travel agent at the time of booking, along with asking about any other requirements you may have.

The following cruise lines and these ships offer a wide selection of special rates, and disabled toilet facilities, disabled cabins with accessible toilets. Pool hoists are also available and special dietary requirements can be easily met. These facilities can be booked in advance through the **North West Cruise Club.**
Helpline: **0161 799 7333**
Website**: www.northwestcruiseclub.co.uk**

Ships Offering Accessible Features and Extra PublicToilet facilities/disabled cabins:

P & O

- Arcadia
- Aurora
- Oceana
- Oriana
- Ventura

Royal Caribbean International

- Adventurer of the Seas
- Explorer of the Seas
- Mariner of the Seas

Celebrity Cruises

- Summit
- Infinity
- Millennium

Fred Olsen

- Boudicca
- Black Prince
- Black Watch

Holland America

- Zuiderdam
- Holland America

Norwegian Cruise Lines (NCL)

- Norwegian Cruise Lines - **All**

MSC Cruises

- Opera

While At Sea

Although no one likes to think of getting sick, especially in the middle of an ocean, it can happen. Cruise ships cannot offer state-of-the-art medical facilities but all shipboard infirmaries must be compliant with the **International Council of Cruise Lines Maritime Medicine Code**. This means that they must provide *reasonable* medical care. Patients requiring serious medical solutions, such as surgical care, will be airlifted to the nearest shore-side facility.

Guidelines also include the requirement for medical staff to be on call twenty-four hours a day, examination and treatment areas, and equipment that includes defibrillators, cardiac monitors, airway equipment, external cardiac pacing, EEG and ECG machines, infusions pumps and a fully stocked emergency cart.

The size of the vessel and the number of passengers determines the composition of the medical staff. Larger cruise ships carry at least two doctors and three nurses. Some innovative ships include live video, voice and data streaming via satellite to land-based specialists who can assist with complex cases. Some ships even carry dialysis machines to enable kidney patients the luxury of a cruise. Some cruise lines also carry on board dentists.

Treatment is chargeable and medical insurance is usually a requirement of booking a cruise. Do refer to the travel insurance companies listed above as cruise companies' own travel insurance will be expensive in view of pre-existing conditions.

Cruise lines do not normally carry ostomy bags so make sure you have an adequate supply. In the event of loss, the cruise line will arrange for supplies to be delivered to the next possible port destination. In an emergency, a sterile rubber glove attached with surgical tape can be used in place of a bag.

Yachting

DR Yachting hosts guests with disabilities and chronic illnesses from all over the world. They consulted with experts in special needs matters, in order to outfit its sailing boats for people needing larger toilet facilities and some disabled features. They have installed a large flat gangway entrance to enable wheelchair access. The bathroom facilities are engineered with ample space to manoeuvre around, and the double-bedded cabins are designed for easy access. The yachts have seat belts on all the seats, and handles are placed around the yacht, to make moving about easy and safe.

Its all-inclusive sailing holidays for people with special needs operate around the Greek Islands, where the year round weather conditions are ideal and the ports have easy access. The yachts are never more than four hours sailing time from one port to the next. They have also installed special safety equipment on board that allows disabled guests to fully participate in and enjoy their vacations on the sea.

DR Yachting can carry to two wheel chair passengers and their companions, or up to eight individuals with various disabilities or chronic illnesses, without compromising

their comfort and dignity. For more information contact:
www.disabledsailingholidays.com
email:**dryachting@hotmail.com**
or Telephone: **30 210 9850168/9**

Useful links for assisted holidays

The following links list holidays for those who need financial help or just accessible (toilet) accommodation. There is a wonderful selection both in the UK and overseas.

3H Fund
www.3hfund.org
Tel: **01892 547 474**

The 3H fund organise group holidays that are subsidised, inclusive of transportation for physically disabled and chronically sick people over eleven years of age.

When funds are available, they also provide grants to families with disabled or chronically sick children to have a modest UK holiday break.

Badaguish Outdoor Centre
www.badaguish.org
Tel: **01479 861 285**

This centre provides a wide range of outdoor activities for physically disabled and chronically sick children. It has a residential holiday unit and 24-hour respite care is available.

Break
www.break-charity.org
Tel: **01263 822 161**

Established in 1968, Break's services include supported holidays, short breaks and day care support for people with learning disabilities, physically disabled and the chronically sick, including self-catering holiday chalets for families with children

Calvert Trust
www.calvert-trust.org.uk
Tel: **020 8405 3826**

For Over thirty years, the Calvert trust has been bringing people with disabilities and chronically sick people, together with abled family and friends to achieve their potential through outdoor activities in the countryside. Its three purpose built centres around the UK offering a wide range of sports and recreational activities. Over 11,000 people annually visit one of the Calvert Centres offering multi breaks and special courses.

Disabled Holiday Directory
www.disabledholidaydirectory.co.uk
This is a wonderful directory of accessible holiday accommodation for disabled and chronically sick and services in the UK, USA, and Europe.

Disabled People's Transport Advisory Committee
www.dptac.gov.uk/door-to-door

This committee studies and advises the UK Government on access to all types of transport for disabled people and people with chronic illness.

The website includes a wealth of information about all kinds of transport, new developments accessible to all and includes details on how to and to whom to complain when things go wrong.

Happy Days Charity
www.happydayscharity.org.uk

Happy Days Is a national children's charity dedicated to providing holidays, days out and theatre trips for disadvantaged young people or children with special needs, chronic or life-limiting illnesses or disabilities.

They will assist children between age three and seventeen. They welcome children from many different backgrounds and cultures and who have many different conditions. They also help young people who have been abused or neglected, witnessed domestic violence, been bereaved or act as carers for a parent or a sibling. In summary, they will provide:

- Holidays for young people and their families

- Days out for groups to hundreds of venues throughout the UK, including the seaside, zoos, theme parks, safari parks and fun fairs.

- Trips to the theatre or shows and theatre workshops

H.E.L.P. (Holiday Endeavour for Lone Parents)
www.helphols.co.uk

Tel: **01427668717**

HELP is a registered charity providing reduced cost holidays for any lone parent and their children, forces wives and children whose husbands are serving abroad. Holidays are available at Haven and Butlin's holiday parks. Special accessible accommodation is available on request. It also owns static caravans at Flamingoland Theme Park and Zoo, Haven Golden Sands, Mablethorpe and Haven primrose Valley at Filey.

HELP representatives are on call at all times. The Government Direct **Payments** scheme can also be used to fund these holidays.

A token membership fee of £5 per year is applied. You may take as many holidays as you wish per year.

Holiday Care
www.holidaycare.org.uk/membership.asp

Livability
www.livability.org.uk

Livability is an organisation supporting disabled and chronically ill people throughout the UK. Besides its care services programmes it offers specialised four* accommodation throughout the UK for disabled and chronically sick. Subsidised pricing is available. However, accommodation can be funded through the John Groom's Charity and the Shaftsbury Society. The Government **Direct Payments** scheme can fund holidays through the Livability organisation that will provide full details on financial help.

National Holiday Fund for Sick and Disabled Children
www.nhfcharity.co.uk
Tel: **01341 280486**

This charity, twinned with a similar charity in the US, provides holidays to Florida for chronically ill children, temporarily or permanently physically disabled children or terminally ill children. Children must be between eight and eighteen.

Each holiday is of two weeks duration with a group normally consisting of twelve children, each of whom is accompanied by a carer. In addition, there is an experienced group leader, a qualified Doctor, a physiotherapist and a senior nurse.

Only hotels, that have been visited and vetted by the N.H.F.'s representatives, are used. All the transport needs for the children of each group are arranged before the holiday.

The children will have the opportunity to enjoy a number of the Orlando theme parks. They will also visit locations and events that have been specially organized by the Charity's USA sister organization.

These may include:

- A trip to Mount Dora on pontoon boats across Lake Dora
- A day at the beach at historic Fort De Soto
- Visits to Gatorland; SeaWorld; Kennedy Space Center; Walt Disney's Magic Kingdom; Epcot; MGM Studio's; Animal Kingdom; Universal Studio's and a Honda motor cycles experience.

Parents, guardians and carers of the children have an opportunity to take a much-needed respite, knowing their charges are having the best of care and continuity of medical attention while they are away from home.

It also provides an opportunity to give extra or undivided attention to others in the family. The heavily subsided cost of these trips is currently £350.00 per child.

Some Grant funding is available to cover the cost from various charitable and indirect government schemes. The NHF will advise on these.

Peter Le Marchant Trust
www.peterlemarchanttrust.co.uk

For over thirty years, this Trust has provided day outings and holidays on waterways for people of all ages with any kind of disability or serious illness.

Unwanted Baggage

The Trust operates three canal boats from its Loughborough base. The season runs from April to October inclusive, every day except Bank Holidays but including weekends. Two boats are available for day outings and one is available for hire for longer periods for people with chronic illnesses and their families. Token charges apply.

Vitalise
www.vitalise.org.uk

Vitalise is a national charity that providing holidays for disabled, chronically sick and visually impaired people and breaks for carers It has been providing short breaks for disabled people, chronically ill patients and carers at accessible Centres in the UK since 1963.

Its centres cater for adults with a variety of disabilities. It aims to provide an alternative to traditional residential respite care. Each centre offers short breaks in a relaxed, holiday style environment with a variety of trips and activities.

Guests on these breaks are supported by volunteers who provide companionship and assistance where and if necessary.

Elizabeth Prosser & Philip Prosser

Accessible Scotland
www.visitscotland.com/guide/where-to-stay/accessible-scotland/

This website is useful if you are planning a holiday in Scotland and have accessibility needs, these include toilet information as well as wheelchair access etc.
On the website, there are a number of options to select accommodation and related lists of activities that are suited to your individual requirements. You must, have a specific destination in mind to use the browsing feature – If this appeared alongside a map of Scotland then it would be ideal, as it is it is difficult to use without a map by your side.

Accessible Wales
www.goodaccesswales.co.uk

The Good Access Guide to Wales is a directory of accessible accommodations, amenities, disabled toilets and disability services.

Through this unique online resource, residents and visitors of all abilities can discover the best in accessible and inclusive living, leisure activities and mobility status.

It includes accessible hotels, cottages, bed and breakfasts, farm stays, caravan parks and inns; museums, theatres, sporting venues, visitor attractions as well as places to wine, dine and generally have a good time.

Unwanted Baggage

RADAR
www.radar.org.uk

RADAR's guide to special need's holidays in Britain and Ireland has been issued for over 30 years. The latest 2010 edition includes detailed information on 1500 places to stay in all parts of the United Kingdom and Republic of Ireland.

It include hotels, guest houses, self-catering cottages and flats, holiday parks, activity centres, campsites and centres where provision is made for specialist services and care. The guide also gives information on advice services, voluntary and commercial organisations and transport. The guide aims to give information that will be useful to people with as wide a range of disabilities as possible.

Choosing your holiday accommodation is made easier by the individual listings stating the size of entrance doors, location of ground floor bedrooms, accessible lifts, and whether there are specially designed bathroom facilities, and if waterproof or feather-free bedding is available

3H Fund
www.3hfund.org.uk

3H Fund organises subsidised group holidays for physically disabled and chronically ill people accompanied by volunteer carers, giving the disabled person a chance to have a unique and enjoyable experience, and providing a break from the routine of caring for the carer or family of that person.

Elizabeth Prosser & Philip Prosser

Access At Last
www.accessatlast.com

Access At Last provides a booking service for accessible holiday accommodation and services in Britain and overseas. It is the only website in the world advertising only accommodation with at least one room with a level access shower and accessible toilet.

Accessible Travel and Leisure
www.accessibletravel.co.uk

This tour operator specialises in accessible holidays all over the world. Their staff will advise you on the suitability of each destination and tailor a holiday to meet specific requirements. Whether you need to ensure ground floor accommodation, handrails, en-suite bathrooms, or any other special facilities, they will secure the most appropriate accommodation and services.

Enable holidays
www.enableholidays.com

Whenever and wherever you would like to go, Enable will help you to see more of the world. Enable Holidays can help you find, plan and arrange a holiday to suit your individual needs Each resort, hotel and apartment featured in their brochure has been carefully assessed to ensure it is accessible and suitable for travellers with any special needs. They will also make any arrangements you may require for the airport, flights and transfers to the resort.

Tourism For all
www.tourismforall.org.uk

Tourism for All UK is a national charity dedicated to making tourism welcoming to all. In the past, there have been difficulties for some wishing to participate in tourism - those with disabilities, chronically sick, older people, and carers of young people or people with accompanying disabled or older relatives - Tourism for All works to overcome these.

On the website, they offer information on where you can stay or visit. They offer advice and assistance to both businesses and public bodies who need to make changes to become more accessible. They have special information on accessible toilets and publish independent special offers on holidays and information in equipment hire abroad.

Away from it all Holidays - AFIA
http://www.themothersunion.org/communitywork.aspx
The Mothers' Union
24 Tufton Street
LONDON SW1P 3RB
Tel: 020 7222 5533
E-Mail: outreach@themothersunion.org

The Mothers' Union is a Christian organisation supporting the institution of family life. Away From It All (AFIA) is a holiday scheme funded by members of the Mothers' Union to help people experiencing stressful situations who would not otherwise be able to have a holiday.

Anyone can apply for a holiday, with each applicant being asked to provide a letter of referral from a professional who knows the family, a GP, social worker, cleric etc.

The holidays provided take many different forms, including caravan holidays, chalet accommodation and family holiday sites. Further details are available on request. Anyone interested in applying should write, in the first instance, to the above address.

Dave Lee's Happy Holidays
www.happyholidays.moonfruit.com
15 Curtis Wood Park Road
HERNE Kent
CT6 7TY
Tel: 01227 371022 – hotline: 01227 728240

This is rather an unusual charity in that it <u>only benefits families who are resident in Kent</u>. The charity organises holidays for disabled, sick and underprivileged children and their immediate families.

Harriet Davis Seaside Holiday Trust
www.harriet-davis-trust.brecon.co.uk
1 Bryncelyn Way
Llangynidr
CRICKHOWELL
Powys NP8 1LY
Tel: 01874 730500

This charity is set up to establish self-catering holiday homes for families with disabled and chronically sick children. Four superb properties are available in Tenby,

Pembrokeshire; all are fully adapted and equipped with a variety of special aids and equipment. One of the houses offers a small indoor heated swimming pool.

Part-time family helpers are employed as necessary. Out of the main holiday season, or if the properties are free, they are also available to disabled or chronically sick adults and their carers. Full details and booking forms are available from the above address or website.

There is a charge for this accommodation, but it is much lower than commercial rates. Other schemes are available to help cover the cost.

Scout Holiday Homes Trust
www.scoutbase.org.uk/hq-info/holhomes
Gilwell Park
Chingford
LONDON E4 7QW
Tel: 020 8433 7100/020 8433 7290

The Trust has specially adapted, fully stocked caravans and chalets at 12 sites in popular locations in England and Wales. Families with a disabled or chronically ill child are most welcome and they do not need to have any connection with scouting.

Most of the accommodation is for up to six people and prices range from £95-£380/week, depending on location and time of year. Every holiday booked this year receives a £10 voucher off any holiday booked for next year, and there is a £25 reduction on second weeks. A Brochure is available from the above address.

Elizabeth Prosser & Philip Prosser

Kids' Days Out
www.kidsdaysout.co.uk/

This is a good directory of accessible children's attractions around the U.K. It includes all the information that you need to plan a successful trip. The guide is broken down into specific areas, counties etc. and includes activities for children alone (supervised) and family groups.

From ceramic painting – to butterfly hatching; from Coasteering (jumping off cliffs)-to white water rafting and animal parks galore – this detailed guide is an excellent resource for all.

Chapter Fourteen
Appliances and Accessories
...All the essentials on bags and necessary extras

If you have a permanent ostomy, you are exempt from prescription costs for the duration of the time you have the Stoma. To apply for the exemption certificate you need to fill in form P11, available from GP or your local Health authority. Many UK based companies will ship overseas for UK pension holders or UK residents. Prescription costs are not currently (2010), applicable in Wales or Scotland

Most stoma necessities are available on the NHS. You can obtain a prescription in the normal way through your GP and local chemist or you can order on-line, or over the telephone from specialised postage-free suppliers or direct from the manufacturers. They will process your prescriptions for you without you needing to contact the surgery or GP. It is a matter of personal choice. You do not have to use any company or service that you are not happy with.

You can change suppliers whenever you want to, to whomever you want. If you prefer, you can also opt for multiple suppliers of different items as well. If you are unhappy with the service you get, (impolite customer service operatives, later deliveries, incorrect deliveries etc.) complain! If you do not get a satisfactory result, change to another company. There is a lot of competition and a high standard of service is expected.

If you opt for a chemist, you must first visit your GP to obtain a prescription. You may find delays in obtaining some items, as they do not carry these as standard and have to order them in themselves from wholesalers and manufacturers. They do not supply the extra free items that are included by suppliers or manufacturers

If you order directly from a manufacturer or supply house, they usually deliver within 48 hours. They will also take care of your prescriptions that will save visits to your GP. Deliveries arrive in discreet plain boxes and these will be left at a designated location if you are not at home. All supply houses provide free carrying bags, wet and dry wipes, water sprays and many other handy specialised items. You can order by email, website, mail or telephone. Twenty-four hour, seven-day-a-week ordering is usually available. This is not usually available through local chemists or GPs.

Everyone has a personal preference – but bear in mind that the larger the organisation, the more anonymous you may be to them .Smaller companies tend to designate a personal contact who will call you regularly to remind you that you are due to re-order and tell you about new products.

Larger companies have nurse advisers that can be helpful if you are unable to reach your own stoma nurse. You may also wish to choose a company local to you – the options are tremendous, and I have indicated my own product preferences. However, I do want to make it clear that ***I have not received any endorsement or funding to do so.***

No two people prefer the same items; *indeed,* I encourage everyone to try each different manufacturer's products to find the ones that suit them best.

Bags – the basics

There are dozens of different pouches/bags available to ostomists today. The first few that you are issued in hospital will seem very large but it will not be long before you are able to test and eventually choose the best manufacturer, size and shape that are right for you. I recommend that you "test drive" as many, different bags as possible, wearing each variety for at least a week to give them a thorough trial before making a final decision.

Keep in mind that your stoma will change throughout your life as well and each change may require a different type of bag or another manufacturer. All Bags come in boxes provided with loose stick-on filter covers that mask the smell. However, if you cover the filter then the trapped wind will not pass out of the bag and may cause ballooning. I recommend leaving these covers off unless you notice an unpleasant smell (This will be caused by odour producing foods).

One of the most important factors is how your skin (around the stoma) will react to the various adhesives that manufacturers use. Even though you may not have suffered allergies in the past, your skin may react to some adhesives, especially after long-term use, - becoming sore, tender and red after an overnight application. You do not have to put up with these skin irritations. You can test as many bags as you wish, until you find the ones that produce little or no irritation.

Nothing need go to waste while you are testing bags to your satisfaction. Any bags and accessories that you have not used can be donated to overseas' charities where any bags are difficult to obtain. The two UK based charity-forwarding groups are:

Jacobs well appeal
2 Ladygate
Beverley
East Yorkshire HU17 8BH
Email: **thejacobswell@aol.com**

Alternatively:

SCAR
Maggie Littlejohn
1B Redburg Gate
Kilwinning Road
Irvine KA12 8TH
Email: **maggielittlejohn@aol.com**

Unwanted Baggage

The main bag choices are as follows:

Clear or discreet?

- **Beige coloured (opaque)** – This bag has a discreet covering to hide the contents. These sometimes have a flap so that you can position the bag correctly.

OR

- **Clear** - These bags are completely transparent– these are usually issued in hospitals so that staff can easily monitor the contents immediately after surgery. Patients sometimes prefer these so they can see at a glance when a bag needs changing.

You can then choose between a:

- **Closed** bag – this bag is completely sealed and has to be changed when it is full. There are now flushable closed bags that can be popped straight into the toilet, especially handy for travelling. (New Easy-Peel™ FreeStyle Vie® Flushable from Clinimed)

OR

- **Open (or flapped) bag** - this has a drain at the neck (bottom) to empty and re-seal. These bags can be kept on for twenty four-forty eight hours before changing. If the skin begins to feel sore or painful, it may be an indication of leakage, in which case change it immediately.

The next choice is either:

- **A one-piece drainable bag** (as above)

OR

- **A two-piece bag** This bag comes with a separate base plate on to which it can be clipped. If you suffer from frequent skin irritations, this bag will allow you to leave the base plate on, while you empty a drainable attachment or change a closed attachment. The base plate can remain for up to four or five days. Extra attention should be give to cleaning the skin under the base plate upon removal to cut down on the build up of bacteria, which can form from any leakage. It is essential to ensure that a base plate forms a tight seal with your skin.

You cannot mix and match base plates and bags from different manufacturers as they are designed to fit exactly.

Body and stoma shapes are different. You can opt for a:

- **Bag with a flat adhesive plate** – This depends on where your stoma is. It is better suited If you are lucky to have it sited on an area of smooth skin or if the stoma extrudes well.

OR

- **A convex bag has a raised centre plate** to accommodate natural skin folds or retracted stomas.

- There are **small closed catchment bags** for short-time use such as bathing, swimming or intimate moments

Dependent upon manufacturer, ostomy bags are made in different length sizes (usually small, medium and large), that you can alternate for different occasions or simply for preference. My personal favourite bag manufacturer is *"Pelican"* as I find their adhesive to be very mild on the skin and, as a smaller company, their ordering team is very helpful and friendly. Again, I encourage you to try a number of different manufacturers' products to find the adhesive that suits you.

The hole in the central base plate in all bags can be cut to size by the manufacturer using a template provided by you or supply you with one of their standard hole sizes (2mm apart). This is your decision, the stoma will change during your lifetime and it must be measured regularly using the guide supplied in each box of bags. If in doubt, ask your stoma nurse to measure and make a template for you. If you wish, you can cut any bag to your preferred size.

A base plate with a hole that is too small may cause the bag to burst and/or leak. A hole that is too large will cause inflammation because of the output acidic/alkaline matter being exposed to the skin around the stoma. If you stoma recedes, then you must use a convex plate. The more it protrudes the better delivery will be into a flat bag.

As your stoma will change in size and shape quite dramatically over the first six months , it is important to measure frequently before re-ordering and to order only two boxes at a time, keeping a reserve box just in case of diarrhoea or other emergency. Most boxes contain thirty bags.

Paediatric and neonatal bags with printed patterns are available from most suppliers.

Due to the frequency of emptying, urostomy bags are drainable and they are fitted with a small soft tap to drain at your convenience. There are no closed urostomy bags. There is a wonderful collection by different manufacturers. Your choice should be based on the adhesive that suits you best. There is also a selection of different sizes.

Prescription accessories:

All the following items are available on prescription:

- **Bag Covers:** - These wonderful items reduce any rubbing between the bag and skin. The majority are made in soft cotton and, from personal experience, really make a difference. These come in a variety of styles and patterns and one manufacturer makes a waterproof cover for that extra protection while bathing

Unwanted Baggage

or swimming. I use **Bullen**'s bag covers because their turnaround time is faster than any others. The bags are made to fit your own ostomy bag come, as standard, in a large variety of patterns/plain/children's etc. They also make the only waterproof covers available in the UK.

You can also provide them with your preferred material. Of course, you can make your own bag covers by using your preferred bag as a guideline. Simply trace the outline onto greaseproof paper and use a second outline to include a base plate gap and an emptying flap. Strips of Velcro hold the bag cover to the base plate.

Several American manufacturers have much larger varieties of patterns and materials including Lycra and towelling. Most of these will export to the UK but these cannot be ordered on prescription. Average cost is about $9-15 per bag cover, plus postage costs.

- **Belts:** – These narrow elasticated belts attach to the loops of a bag giving added security.

- **Stoma cups:** – These hard cups protect ostomates who play active sports or are involved in heavy lifting etc.

- **Corsets & Underwear:** - You can order six pairs of specialised underpants with a pocket designed to hold the bag in basic styles by getting a prescription from your GP and sending this to your preferred manufacturer or supplier. Specialised corsets that allow for the bag's expansion and contain a pocket are also available.

Lotions and potions on prescription

There are many creams, lotions, pastes, gels and adhesive plates that help to make life easier. I have indicated those I personally use, although I encourage you to try all the different manufacturer's products as everyone reacts differently to scents/adhesives/content etc. Details of these, all available on prescription, are as follows:

- **Flanges:** – these sit on top of the bag to hold it more firmly in place. The adhesive is stronger and more aggressive than normal bag standard adhesive and can cause skin irritation. I am currently using **Second Nature. Nature secuPlast circular plasters** as these are a one-piece ring that is so easy to use. It can also be cut, using pieces to secure areas that are more susceptible to leakage. I also like the *SecuPlast hydrocolloid secuPlast* although the packaging is awkward as once opened all the strips tend to fall out. I repackage them into an ordinary plastic bag for use.

- **Adhesive plates, rings, and tapes:** – these can be used under or over the bag, onto the base plate. If they are used under the bag, then the bag can be applied to them adding a double layer of adhesive. (The adhesive is slightly more aggressive which could cause skin irritation). Plates need to be cut to size

Unwanted Baggage

allowing for the stoma opening. Adhesive tapes are easy to use to secure the bag. I prefer the ***Bullen flange retention strips.*** These really stick well and cannot be removed without an adhesive remover. As for rings, if a convex bag is not convex enough for those people with inverted stomas, either the **Eakin's or Pelican's washers** are great and the adhesive is a lot milder than other washer adhesives.

- **Paste:** - this is a difficult product to use, no matter which manufacturer you choose. However, if all else fails, it is the answer to severe leakage. It is used to fill scarring or skin folds to assist in forming a very tight seal. This is very effective but rather messy and has a long drying time while you wait to replace the bag. While waiting for the paste to set, cover the stoma with a cotton swab to catch leaking matter. Use disposable gloves or you will spend an inordinate amount of time trying to get the paste off your hands.

- *Do not use paste unless you have a two-piece bag or plan on leaving your bag on for at least 48 hours.* The best paste remover is Pelican's Citrus Adhesive Remover. Use only tepid water and soap to remove the residue thereafter. For my own use, I found Eakin's paste to be the most effective and the least irritating to the skin. For all pastes, adequate Instructions on how to use pastes are not included in the manufacturer's packaging

– if you have any problems with either applying or removing paste, telephone the manufacturers (in Eakin's case, as a novice paste user, they were fantastically responsive – even telephoning back on a Saturday to make sure I was able to remove the paste successfully).

- **Adhesive remover:** – this comes in wipes (sachets) and aerosol spray form. I use the aerosol to remove the bag and the wipe to remove any excess adhesive before washing the stoma site. I prefer the ***Appeel®*** and ***Trio's Niltac™*** sprays and ***Pelican Citrus Adhesive Remover*** sachets for heavy-duty removal (pastes, rings, flanges, tapes etc.) and ***Appeel®*** adhesive removal sachets for basic bag adhesive removal.

- **Barrier cream/gel/spray/sachet:** – These products offer additional protection to the skin prior to the application of the bag. You must wait until the barrier has dried before applying the bag. Barrier cream comes in multi format types: Creams and gels both of which take a little longer to dry before you can apply the bag; sachet wipes that evaporate quickly and sprays that dry very quickly. I like the ***LBF® No Sting Barrier sachets***, pressing the whole wipe over the area where the bag sits; once it has dried (seconds). The new added **vitamin E barrier film by Pelican** is also very good. I then apply the ***3M Spray Cavilon™ No sting Barrier Film*** for extra protection.

Unwanted Baggage

- **Powders:** - These powders are useful to dry any parts that are bleeding or sore within the exposed stoma ring. Slight bleeding is very normal inside the stoma ring and on skin immediately around the stoma. I have found that the best way to apply this is to pour a small pinch into my hand and use a cotton bud to apply directly to the affected area. My personal preference is the ***Ostoseal™ Aloe Vera Protective Powder****as you can apply it under the bag's adhesive area.*

- **Odour control sprays:** – These can be sprayed over the toilet after emptying the bag and come in many varieties and manufacturers. You cam also spray a little directly into the bottom of the bag. I like the ***OstoMist Odour Neutraliser*** – the "Cinnamon & Sandalwood" scent lingers for quite a while and is ozone friendly. The **OstoZyme Gel** is excellent for odour control and can be easily popped into the neck (bottom) of the bag as you change appliances.

- **Output Thickeners**: – These are generally for ileostomates, as their faecal output tends to be liquid. These come in a variety of types, - sachets, pills placed into the bag – all work equally well although I find the ***Diamond™ sachets*** are very good for extreme liquid output but can emit a fine black powder onto your hands as you handle them. The ***Absorbian Wands*** by ***Bullen*** are great for lighter use for both colostomates with a slight liquid problem and continual use for ileostomates. The new **Pelican Perform** solidifying sachets are also proving an excellent product for medium output product and are clean to use.

- **Pancake Prevention:** – Pancaking is a common problem for colostomates. It will cause leakage and bursting if left unattended. Initially, you will feel a small build up in the bag around the stoma. Manually massage the top of the bag from the outside to push the content down. If this is a regular problem then there is a new product on the market to help. This is a *"Stoma Bridge Clearway"* – which can be inserted at the top of the bag through the base plate hole. Produced by **Opus Healthcare,** this is a long awaited, much needed and unique product! **Ostozyme gel** also helps to stop pancaking if popped into an empty bag before its application and then massaged to ensure it covers the whole bag. Another alternative is to pop a few drops of baby oil into the bag when you empty it. Do not apply baby oil into a bag that is unattached, as it can cause leakage problems to the adhesive around the stoma.

- **Disposal Bags, wet and dry wipes etc.:** – You will find that a number of ancillary, complimentary products are also included at in your order. These vary from the different suppliers/manufacturer and they will normally ask you how many of each you require and supply these as courtesy products. Your first order will also contain special cases that are especially designed with compartments to hold several bags, and accessories for a few changes.

Disposal bags are essential, as you **must not flush bags** in the toilet. (There are flushable inserts but these are difficult to fit into place inside a bag after removing the old one although most main drainage companies ask that these not be flushed down the toilet anyway!). One bag is usually sufficient to hold all the wipes and swabs you use during changing. Once sealed, they can be disposed of with general household refuse. Several councils will provide you with a small yellow chemical waste disposal bin if their local rules demand it. (See council's policy on nappies). ***Wet and Dry wipes*** are essential to clean the stoma and surrounding areas and protect skin/clothes while changing/emptying. The wet wipes are similar to baby wipes but are medically approved.

In addition to these, I also order prescription item **CliniMed®'s woven swabs** in packs of 100 as I find these very useful to contain faecal matter that oozes whilst you are cleaning. No matter what you do, the stoma has a mind of its own and there is no way to predict its output but you can guarantee that it will definitely ooze whilst changing the bag!

Elizabeth Prosser & Philip Prosser

Be Prepared!

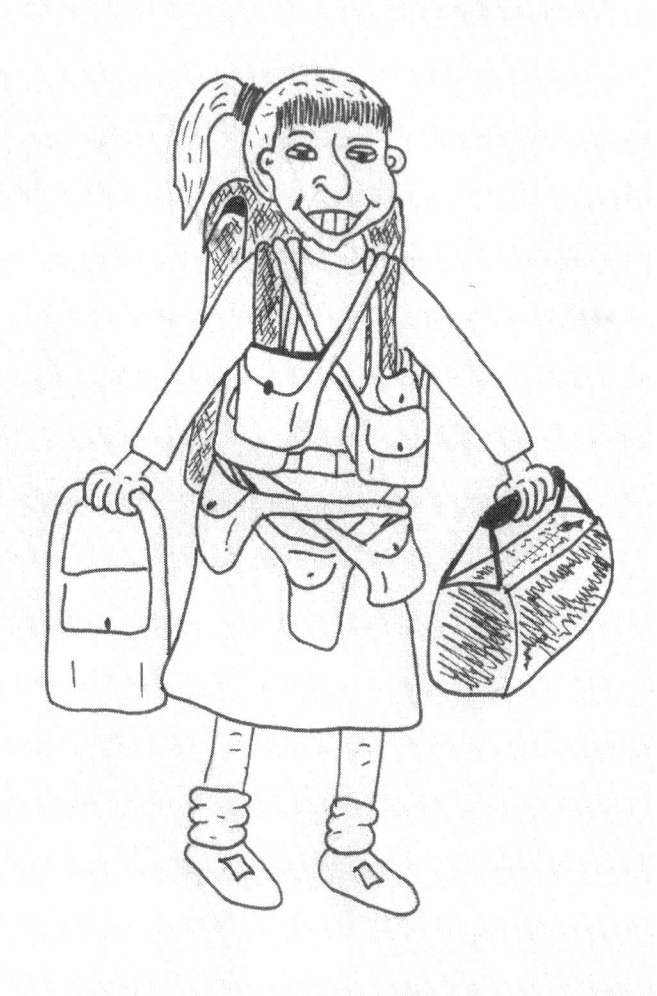

The following is a comprehensive list of UK suppliers and manufacturers:

Some manufacturers/suppliers details may have changed since publication and the author/publisher cannot be held responsible for any incorrect information listed below.

AlphaMed Ltd   Supplier
Ostomy & Urostomy products
Day Lewis House,
340 Bensham Lane,
Thornton Heath Surrey
CR7 7EQ
Tel:: **0800 515317**
Email: **sjames@alphamed.co.uk**
www.alphamed.co.uk

AlphaMed specialises in the safe, secure and discreet delivery of stoma care and continence products throughout the UK. It offers a free, first class delivery service direct to your door-by courier of a range of stoma supplies.

Amcare Ltd   Supplier
Ostomy & Urostomy products
Also agents for Convatec (Bag Manufacturer)
Unit 69, Riverside 3
Sir Thomas Longley Rd
Medway City Estate
Strood
Kent
ME2 4BH
Freephone: **0800 885050**

Email: **amcare.order@bms.com**
www.convatec.co.uk/amcare/services/nursing.html

Amcare™ is the stoma care home delivery service arm of **ConvaTec** (bag manufacturer) It has a reputation for a fast, efficient and caring service that has been serving the ostomate community for almost 20 years.

Supplies any ostomy product upon request.
Its own specialist products include:

- girdles for stoma hernias and specialised fitting service
- Nurse advisory Team
- Support cushions for post surgery recovery

Am Care has a network of twelve local care centres, each with a team of dedicated helpers and regular delivery couriers to make sure you get your stoma supplies as promptly and discreetly as possible.

BetterCare   Supplier
Ostomy underwear and filter
BetterCare BV
Kade 51
4703 GC Roosendaal
Netherlands
Tel: **00-31 165 55 59 02** (NL)
email: **info@bettercare.nl**
www.bettercare.nl

Bettercare is the European distributor for two ostomy products. These are available for export by ordering

Unwanted Baggage

by email or telephone. English speakers operate the telephone ordering line.

- Unique "Wear-close" is bag combination cover/panty especially designed to wear under bathing costumes or close fitting garments. Available in a variety of colours, designed for wearing on either side of the body. Soft breathable material.

- Osto–EZ-Vent designed especially for patients who experience extreme wind build up and for ostomy airline travellers. This unique gadget fits on any bag and works to remove any excess wind, eliminating bag bursting etc.

Braun Medical Ltd **Manufacturer**
Ostomy & Urostomy products
Thorncliffe Park
Sheffield
Tel. **0114-225 9000**
Email:**customercare.bbmuk@bbraun.co.uk**
www.bbraun.co.uk

B. Braun UK is a global manufacturer of a full range of medical products. It manufactures urostomy and ostomy bags and accessories that must be ordered through a supplier. It does not supply directly but is happy to provide samples on request.

The website is a good information source for all its products. Braun products are available from all suppliers.

Specialist Products:

- Softima® One Piece Ostomy Bags - available as a Drainable (Flow Control) and closed pouch.
- Carisoft® cleansing pads
- Biotrol®– skin protection plate – various sizes
- Biotrol® capsules for neutralising odour (in-bag)
- Alymarys® stoma adjustable belts
- B.Braun Ileo Gel – gel bag tablets for absorbing fluids (for ileostomates).

Brunlea Surgical   Supplier
Ostomy & Urostomy products
Freepost unit 10, Balderstone close
Burnley
Lancashire
BB10 1BR.
Freephone: **0800 834712**
E-mail:**info@brunleasurgical.co.uk**
www.brunleasurgical.co.uk

Brunlea is a family business, established in 1983, offering a personal door-to-door service of Colostomy and Incontinence products to the **NW area** by their own delivery vans. They also offer same-day delivery on orders received before 11:30am. They have excellent connections with local hospitals and stoma nurses in the area.

Unwanted Baggage

Product Range:

- Full range of stoma appliances and accessories
- Full range of Ostomy bags – Urostomy bags
- Bag Covers
- Belts
- Irrigation supplies
- Incontinence and Urostomy supplies
- Catheters
- Swabs
- Tapes
- Dressings
- Free toiletry bag/wipes and disposal bags.

BullenHealthcare **Manufacturer/Supplier**
Ostomy & Urostomy products
85-87 Kempston Street
Liverpool, L3 8HE
Telephone: **0151 207 1239**
Freephone : **0800 269327**
Email: **info@bullens.com**
www.bullens.com

Bullen Healthcare Group is a fourth generation, family-run company established in 1858. Its personalised Home Delivery Service provides the delivery of the full range of stoma products and prescription appliances and accessories to Ileostomists, Colostomists and Urostomists across the whole of the UK.

Their friendly and dedicated team will call you regularly to check your product levels and make sure your requirements are delivered within your desired timeframe. Bullen

Healthcare is happy to deliver **any make or manufacturer of product**. They also manufacture and distribute a range of specialist products and accessories that many people find useful:

Bullen's Specialist Products:

- **Trio Niltac** – this Silicone Medical Adhesive Remover comes in both a spray and in wipes. This product enables the quick, easy and pain free removal of all pouches every time.

- **Trio Silesse** – this Silicone Skin Barrier is available in a soft pump spray and in wipes. This skin care product helps to maintain skin integrity and reduce trauma caused by adhesives.

- **Trio Diamonds** – these sachets are double action, as they not only act as a highly effective discharge-solidifying agent but they also help to alleviate all odour.

- **Absorbian Range** – these discharge solidifying agents come in a range of wands and sachets to suit all of the possible requirements of ostomates.

- **SafeSeals** – these curved hydrocolloid strips provide the ostomate with peace of mind and security from leaks.

- **Bullen's retention slips** - waterproof strips that can be cut to size

Unwanted Baggage

- **Bullen's Bag Covers** - these are available in children's and adult's patterns and a waterproof variety. They make wearing a bag so much more comfortable.

- **Bullen girdles** - these come in a variety of styles and are made to measure.

- **Carefix Stomasafe** Support Garment – this amazing product is designed to offer security and peace of mind to ostomates and disguises the fact that you are wearing a bag – it is incredibly lightweight and easy to slide on. It is available in S, M, L, XL sizes. However, beware of the sizing. The Small size is suitable for an eight-ten year old average **child.** Medium is Ladies size 8-10; Large is Ladies size 12-14; Extra Large is Ladies size 16-18. (Suitable for small man).

- **Shelter Pouches** – Bullen Healthcare have recently launched a new range of Colostomy and Ileostomy bags and provide a full range of bags for newborn through to infants and on to adults, providing appliances to suit all needs.

As part of **Bullen Healthcare's Home Delivery Service,** it also offers absorbent mattress protectors, absorbent bed pads, disposal bags, and wet and dry wipes all **free of charge** to all ostomates using their service.

On a personal note, Bullen's provide an excellent home delivery service, their customer care telephone team

are friendly and helpful. I especially love their bag covers and cannot manage without them!

Linda Butler Bag Covers Manufacturer
Bag Covers
Telephone: 01205 723327

Manufactures bag covers using your own material or supplies wonderful designs. Not available on prescription

Charter Healthcare   Supplier
Ostomy, Urostomy & wound care products
Charter Healthcare
Peterborough Business Park
Peterborough
Cambs. PE2 6FX
Freephone: **0800 132 787**
Email: **gbccare@charter-healthcare.co.uk**
www.charterhealthcare.co.uk

Charter Healthcare provides all Stoma Care products, Continence Care and Wound Care products delivered discreetly to your door. It is primarily an agent for the Coloplast range of products in the UK. It supplies all makes of bags and accessories to the whole of the UK.

- All products are delivered to the door in completely unbranded packaging by a standard high street courier.

- Your exact measurements will be scanned for labels to be produced each time you order, so that the cutting remains precise time after time.

Unwanted Baggage

- **Charter** – a unique periodic magazine for its customers

Specialised Range of Products:

- Full Coloplast range of ostomy bags
- Belts
- Deodorants
- Filters/bridges
- Irrigation washout appliances
- 1& 2 piece urostomy bags
- Full range of urostomy products and accessories
- Irrigation products and accessories

CliniMed Ltd – SecuriCare   Supplier
Ostomy & Urostomy products
Cavell House, Knaves Beech Way
High Wycombe
Bucks HP10 9QY
Freephone: **0800 0360100**
Email: **enquiries@clinimed.co.uk**
www.clinimed.co.uk

CliniMed® markets and distributes Stoma Care , Urology and Continence products among other surgical needs. Its range includes:

In particular, the FreeStyle Vie model has a new soft backing and FreeStyle Flushable is the world's leading flushable colostomy pouch.

Accessories include the excellent no-sting skin care products: LBF barrier wipes and Appeel adhesive removers that make stoma pouch changing even easier whilst also protecting sensitive skin. Suitable for both ostomates and urostomates.

CliniMed distributes Instillagel that is used widely by health professionals in hospitals and in the community. **BioDerm** , a unique male continence device and **CliniFix** - its new skin friendly tube fixation device.

Coloplast Ltd   Manufacturer
Ostomy & Urostomy products
Peterborough Business Park
Peterborough
Cambs.
PE2 6FX
Tel: **01733-39 20 00**
www.coloplast.co.uk

Coloplast Limited is a wholly owned subsidiary of Coloplast A/S of Denmark. Coloplast is the sales, marketing and distribution arm for Coloplast Stoma Care, Wound Care and Continence Care products for the United Kingdom and Eire.

An amazing 40-year history of revolutionary technology allowed the production of the first ever-plastic ostomy pouch in the industry. Charter Healthcare is the direct supplier for Coloplast and other stoma and continence care companies' products directly to users

Product Ranges & Services:

- **Assura** bags
- **Easiflex** bags

Unwanted Baggage

Sensura bags
Accessories
(Creams etc) including **OAD** a very effective appliance deodorant
Charter
- Free Quarterly Ostomy Magazine produced by Charter Healthcare on behalf of coloplast.

<u>Comfizz Ltd</u>   Manufacturer
Clothing
Birkin House
Haddlesey Road
Birkin
Knottingley
WF11 9LT
Telephone: **01757 229 531**
<u>www.comfizz.com</u>

Comfizz is a family business established in 1998 as a Specialised Garment Design and Manufacturer with experience in the textile & clothing industry they know about fabrics and fashions. With its in-house design service it can put together great ideas with the latest fabrics to create any garment you can conceive.

Comfizz understands the need to feel 'normal' after surgery. Nobody wants to be reminded about being different by having to wear 'medical' garments. Comfizz™ Stoma and Hernia Support Wear <u>briefs</u> , <u>boxers</u> and <u>waistbands</u> help fulfil that need. The good thing about these products is that they are **<u>available on prescription</u>**. Ladies styles are however very basic, but the fabric is excellent.

ConvaTec Ltd Manufacturer
Ostomy & urostomy products
Harrington House, Milton Road
Ickenham, Uxbridge UB10 8PU
Freephone: **0800 289738**
www.convatec.co.uk

ConvaTec was founded in 1978 based on two products designed to improve the quality of life for ostomates.

One of the initial products, Stomahesive skin barrier, was a remarkable improvement over the original existing methods of protecting the skin around the stoma. Stomahesive skin barrier led to another major innovation - the Sur-Fit system.

For the first time, people with ostomies could change their ostomy pouches without having to remove the adhesive wafer around the stoma every time, creating the first two-piece system

Some of ConvaTec's Latest Products and Services:

- Esteem synergy
- Natura
- Accessories
- Stomahesive Paste

Covercare Manufacturer
Bag Covers
Tel: 01773 536816

Manufactures a line of cotton bag covers – not on prescription.

Unwanted Baggage

CUI Wear   Manufacturer
Clothing& underwear
CUI International Ltd,
FREEPOST NAT3363
Leicester LE8 4BZ
Freephone: 0800 279 2050
www.cuiwear.com

CUI WEAR is owned by **CUI International**, a leading healthcare company specialising in medical garments for incontinence, ostomy and hernia support. Many of their garments are available on prescription.

- Knickers, Camis and Swimwear for ladies
- Underwear and swim shorts for men

Dansac   Manufacturer
Ostomy & Urostomy products
James Hall, St Ives Business Park
Parsons Green, St Ives
Cambridgeshire
PE27 4AA
Freephone: **0800 581117**
www.dansac.co.uk

Dansac is an international company that develops and manufactures stoma care products. Dansac minis are excellent for swimming, showering or bathing!!

Dansac, founded in 1971 in Fredensborg, Denmark, is part of the Hollister group and has its head office is in Chicago, Illinois, USA.

Elizabeth Prosser & Philip Prosser

Some of Dansac Product Range:
Dansac mini pouch (which I have recommended)
NovaLife2 unique flushable bags (new)
Full range of ostomy and urostomy bags and accessories
Dansac and Hollister sponsors www. C3life.com forum for ostomy users. This has many interesting articles, comments and Utube videos Great forum!!

<u>Farnhurst Medical Ltd</u>   **Supplier**
Ostomy & Urostomy products
Unit 11, Alfold Craft Centre
Alfold
Surrey
GU6 HAP
Freephone: **0800 833876**
email: **info@farnhurst-medical.co.uk**
<u>www.farnhurst-medical.co.uk</u>

Farnhurst is a family run business with commitment to care. It has first hand experience of Stoma Care and a vast knowledge of Ostomy Appliances ensuring confidence and peace of mind.

Farnhurst Specialist services: **CAREFREE HOLIDAY SERVICE:** Farnhurst Medical will dispatch your appliances in advance of your arrival, anywhere in the UK upon your request. They will also re-pack your supplies in easy to carry packets, based on customs and excise specifications, for those trips abroad.

Other appliances: It supplies a wide variety of other appliances including

- hernia belts
- catheters
- sheaths,
- Vacuum therapy products - Osbon Medical, Genesis Medical, Owen-Mumford, Farnhurst-Elite etc.

Fittleworth Medical Ltd   Supplier
Ostomy & Urostomy products
Unit L, Rudford Industrial estate
Ford, Arundel
West Sussex
BN18 0BD
Freephone: **0800 378846**
www.fittleworth.net

Fittleworth is an independent supplier of all ostomy products. It is also the UK agent for **Hollister products.**
In over 20 years, it has built an enviable reputation for reliable delivery and discreet service. Its thirteen care centres provides a large and flexible stock, ensuring essential product availability and offering local delivery.
Its unique service, **World Assist Alliance** - Delivering an easier lifestyle for tourists and travellers. This service allows Fittleworth customers to help you with an emergency supply of appliances and accessories in most overseas locations. The service is free and is combined with specialist nursing advice, as needed in situ. It avoids the need for prescriptions or insurance claims.

Homecare   Supplier
Ostomy & Urostomy products
62 Oak Hill Trading Estate
Worsley Road North

Elizabeth Prosser & Philip Prosser

Walkden
Manchester
M28 5PT
Freephone: **0800 243 103**

General distributor for bags and accessories. **No website**. Local deliveries only.

Hollister   **Manufacturer**
Ostomy & Urostomy products
Hollister products are only available through its UK distributor, Fittleworth (see above)
www.hollister.com/uk

Hollister Limited is dedicated to delivering the highest standard of products and services in *Ostomy Care* and *Continence Care*. Each of its product lines is backed by a policy of unconditional customer satisfaction and each member of the Hollister team is committed to making a difference in the lives of people who use its products.

Specialist Products:

- Moderna flex – ostomy &urostomy bags
- Conform ostomy & urostomy bags
- Impression ostomy & urostomy bags
- Flanges
- Skin fillers and protectives.
- Hollister Skin Care Accessories
- Adhesives and adhesive removers
- Clamps
- Adjustable ostomy belts.
- Urostomy Night Drainage Bag
- Urostomy Night Drain Tube

Unwanted Baggage

- Urostomy Night Drain Tube Long
- Urostomy Night Drain Tube Adaptor
- Urostomy accessories.
- Irrigation sets.

Independence Products   Manufacturer
Ostomy products
Telephone: 01733 536814
www.independenceproducts.co.uk

Their products are available from your usual suppliers:

- Adhesive Remover - aerosol spray and wipes
- Absorbent strips - convert bag fluid into solid
- Barrier Film - special non-sting formula
- Odour Eliminator   - Pump spray that neutralises odours, unscented.

Intimate Moments Apparel   Manufacturer
Ostomy underwear and lingerie (M&F)
2301 Hemingway Lane, Mahwah, New Jersey 07430
Telephone: **00-1-201-825-9486** (US)
www.intimatemomentsapparel.com

This company exports to the UK but does not accept orders via email. Please telephone orders through to obtain exact postage. Gorgeous, discreet, intimate apparel in silk and lace for ostomy patients. Unique lounging trousers for men (complete with bag pouch). Relatively inexpensive, despite overseas postage.

ISOS Briefly Manufacturer
Clothing/underwear
46 Causeway End
Coupar Angus, Blairgowrie
Perthshire
PH13 9DX
Telephone: **01828 626196**
email: **info@isosbriefly co.uk**
www.isosbriefly.co.uk

Isobel Fury is the designer and creator of specialised clothing and undergarments for those wearing medical appliances.

All products have patented supportive in-built concealed pouches and are all made individually for a perfect fit. Quality is excellent.

Just Gloves Manufacturer/Supplier
Disposable gloves, knickers, aprons etc.
Enefco House
The Quay
Poole
Dorset
BH15 1HJ
Freephone: **0800 1777118**
Email: **sales @justgloves.co.uk**
www.justgloves.co.uk

Just Gloves offers a wide range of disposables. These include gloves – latex and non-latex; disposable underwear; first aid products and sanitisers. The disposable aprons are really useful for bag changes, especially if you have

Unwanted Baggage

to change a bag while wearing business or other special clothes. All products are very reasonably priced.

My Heart Ties — Manufacturer
Silk Bag Covers
5148 Peach Street #335
Erie,
PA 16509
United States
info@myheartties.com

www.myheartties.com
"My Heart Tie" Ostomy Pouch Covers allow women with ostomies to feel beautiful and secure during times of intimacy. This is much more than ostomy camouflage; this is truly beautiful and sexy lingerie! Many women love to wear the My Heart Tie Ostomy Pouch Cover by itself. Others wear it with their own special lingerie. Which Heart Tie will you choose and how will you wear yours? My Heart Tie Ostomy Pouch Covers are created from luxurious and sensual brocade fabrics and silks. Each Heart Tie Ostomy Pouch Cover is beautifully hand sewn and finished by a team of dedicated and talented women in the United States. These are however relatively expensive at **$49.50** each, but are made of pure silk. The company is happy to export to the UK.

Nikris ltd — Manufacturer
Bag Alarm for leakage
Telephone: 01926 815518
email:info@stomalert.co.uk
www.stomalarm.co.uk

Nikris manufactures a unique alarm that clips onto the bag leading to a sensor unit that either vibrates or emits a small sound, enough to wake a sleeping ostomate to warn of imminent leakage or an expanding bag. A Must have for ileostomates especially.!!

<u>Oakmed</u>   Supplier
Ostomy & Urostomy products
54 Adams Avenue,
Northampton,
NN1 4LJ.
Freephone: 0800 592786
<u>www.oakmed.co.uk</u>

Oakmed's Company Aim is to provide the highest quality products and services to all those involved with ostomy and wound care whilst ensuring they are cost effective for the National Health Service. Good Delivery services throughout the UK.

Some of Oakmed's Latest Product's and Services:

- Colostomy
- bags
- Ileostomy
- bags
- Urostomy
- bags
- Stoma Caps
- Accessories

New Product: New Stoma Paste that does not dry out.

Unwanted Baggage

Oh POO   Manufacturer
Bag Covers
www.ohpoo.net

Oh Poo manufactures patented designed bag covers for every occasion. Special designs. Not available on prescription.

Opal-London   Supplier
Emergency underwear
www.opal-london.com

Opal distributes "Pocket Pants", emergency thongs for Girls on the Go!

These spare panties are always useful for ostomates. Flesh, white or black cotton thongs are compressed into a cute heart shape and shrink-wrapped so they take up next to no room in your handbag, glove-box, office drawer, pocket, travel bag, carry-on luggage, briefcase.....
.
Fours designs to choose SMARTY pants!, STOP OUT pants! PICK UP pants! and....PARTY pants! "In case of emergency break seal!"   Great extra pair to carry for ostomates.

OSTOMART   Manufacturer/Supplier
Ostomy & Urostomy products
Unit 1,
The Carlton Business Centre,
Carlton,
Nottingham,
England,
NG4 3AA.

Elizabeth Prosser & Philip Prosser

Freephone: **0800 220 300**
Email Address: **enquiries@ostomart.co.uk**
www.ostomart.co.uk

Ostomart, founded in 1991, is unique in having achieved the ISO2002 for high quality and excellent service. A family run, client oriented company, it devotes a high percentage of its profits to be used to research and develop new products and services.

Product Ranges and Services:

- Osto*Mist* a wonderful odour neutralizing sprays – their new scent is cinnamon and sandalwood!
- Osto*Seal* - a superb protective powder containing aloe vera.
- Osto*Shield* – a hard plastic shield for team sports and heavy-duty work.
- Osto*Guard* – soothing barrier cream.
- Osto**Sorb –** neutralizing gel and sachets.
- Osto**Fix** – security strips to anchor the bags.
- Osto**Clear** - adhesive remover in pump spray and sachet made with tea tree and lavender.
- Osto**Zyme** –an excellent neutralising bag lubrication to prevent pancaking
- Osto**Clenz –** cleansing gel for when washing facilities are unavailable
- **Coversure** – bag covers made-to-measure, limited colours/styles.
- Responder - Home Delivery Service
- Complete Range of bags.

Many more products and services are available on the Ostomart website, including a wide selection of fashionable ostomate-suitable clothing, ranging from male and female swimwear, to underwear, to trousers.

I do love the bag covers and the odour sprays that have long lasting scents!

Ostomy Confidence Manufacturer
Ostomy Belts
275 Wolverine Drive,
Walled Lake,
Michigan 48390
United States
Telephone **00-1-248-438-6655** (US) .
email: **service@ostomyconfidence.com**
www.ostomyconfidence.com

Ostomy Confidence manufactures wonderfully soft belts that hold the bag firmly in place, suitable to wear during intimate moments.

The belts are manufactured in cotton/spandex in multiple sizes suitable for both men and women. Easy On- line ordering also allows its product to be exported to the UK. Please email separately for postage costs.

Marlen Healthcare Manufacturer
/supplier
Ostomy Products
Shell Building
Malt Mill Lane,

Halesowen, B62 8JB
telephone: 0330 555 1250
Email: sales@marlenhealthcare.co.uk
www.marlenhealthcare.co.uk

Founded 50 years ago in Cleveland Ohio, US, Marlen is an international supply company that manufactures **Gemini** bags for all ostomates.

One of its unique products is AquaTack™ Hydrocolloid Barrier. It is the only **CONVEX** hydrocolloid barrier that can be folded in half and then in half again yet still retain its shape on rebound! Its unique properties are:

- Absorbs skin moisture
- Adheres to moist skin
- Seals securely; removes easily from sensitive skin (controlled adhesion)

Pelican Healthcare Manufacturer
/Supplier
Ostomy & Urostomy products
Pelican Healthcare Ltd
Quadrant Centre
Cardiff Business Park
Llanishen
Cardiff
CF14 5WF
Freephone: **0800 052 7471**.
email: **contactus@pelicanhealthcare.co.uk**
www.pelicanhealthcare.co.uk

Pelican Healthcare is an established British company, based in Cardiff, who is committed to the design and manufacture of stoma care appliances. With state-of-

Unwanted Baggage

the-art manufacturing facilities and active research and development, the company has been instrumental in bringing many innovative products to the healthcare market. This, together with a positive input from specialist clinicians and other professional customers, ensures that Pelican Healthcare remains at the forefront of providing clinically and cost effective products.

Pelican Healthcare manufactures a wide range of products to suit all stoma types. Pelican pouches are hypoallergenic and have a unique comfortable and secure skin protector. The Pelican range consists of both a one and two-piece selection of pouches, in both flat and a unique soft convex range. All pouches are available in three sizes. Pelican also offer a Paediatric range that has been specifically created with children in mind. An extensive range of accessories is also available.

Pelican Healthcare products are available either from your usual supplier or through the Pelican Home Delivery that offers a fast, efficient and friendly service. Pelican can supply all prescription stoma care appliances, whether manufactured by Pelican or not and offers many benefits to anyone that joins the service.

New products are in development continually so check the website to see the latest developments.

On a personal note, I have found the Pelican delivery service and all its products to be excellent. The adhesive is particularly good for problem skin.
Speciality Products:

- Select Afresh Closed
- Select Afresh Drainable
- Paediatric & Neonatal
- Citrus Fresh Deodorant
- Pelican Protective Wafers
- Pelican Paste
- Ultra Barrier Cream
- Citrus Fresh Adhesive Remover

Pelican Perform solidifying Agent
New from Pelican:

- Extension of the convex pouch to **60mm.**
- New Release no-sting adhesive remover with **added vitamin E**
- New Release Barrier Cream with **added**
- **Vitamin E**

Salts Medilink Manufacturer/Supplier
Ostomy & Urostomy products
639 Garratt Lane
Earlsfield
London
SW18 4SX
Freephone: **0800 626388**
E-mail: **salt@salts.co.uk**
www.salts.co.uk

Salts Healthcare manufacture and supply stoma care and orthotic products. With offices in the UK, Ireland and mainland Europe, they are one of the oldest family owned ostomy supply companies in the UK. Salts is committed to improving the lives of patients all over the world.

Unwanted Baggage

Bringing family values into their service, they have earned a reputation for being one of the friendliest companies in healthcare.

Specialist products:
- **Dermacol®** is a unique stoma collar that provides a leak proof barrier around the base of the stoma, preventing output from coming into contact with the skin.

- **Harmony® Duo** Launched in 2008, it truly gives patients the best of both worlds. It offers all the advantages of a one-piece, with all the convenience of a two-piece system.

- **Stoma Solutions** - Its range of easy-to-use Stoma Solutions has been specifically developed to alleviate the problems faced by ostomists such as leaks, sore skin, residue, odour, skin protection and adhesion.

SASH Medical Ltd Manufacturer
Supplier
Stoma Belts
Woodhouse Rd
Hockley
Essex
SS5 4RU
Freephone: 08003893111
www.sashstomabelts.com

These belts are deigned by an Ostomist!

- Security & Leakage Belt: These belts are available on prescription, made of soft 23mm elastic belt that attaches to retaining flange.

- Stoma Support & Hernia Belt; this is made from 50mm non-elasticised webbing attached to a restraining flange.

SecuriCare (Medical) Ltd Supplier
Ostomy & Urostomy products
Securicare (Medical) Limited
Compass House
Knaves Beech Way
Loudwater
High Wycombe
Bucks
HP10 9QY
Freephone: **0800 585 125**
email: **enquiries@securicaremedical.co.uk**
www.securicaremedical.co.uk

SecuriCare (Medical) Ltd is an award-winning stoma delivery service that prides itself on a friendly and efficient service to ostomates and those that assist them. It Provides:
- A free home delivery service in the UK for all stoma supplies.

- Specialist stoma care nursing in hospitals and the community.

- A Freephone **Careline** for advice and free samples of all brands of stoma pouches and accessories.

All makes and brands of stoma pouches and accessories are delivered direct to door including Welland, Dansac, Convatec, Coloplast, Pelican and many others. Its modern warehouse stocks all brands of pouches and accessories. Their fast turnover ensures that products are always fresh.

With SecuriCare's free "cut-to-fit" service, the fuss of customising your own flanges is taken away. Its new state-of-the-art cutting machine ensures smooth edges. You can send in your prescription in the special freepost envelopes supplied for delivery within 48 hours **or** they will organise your prescription for you with its 'Golden' service – just make one phone call to request supplies and they will collect your prescription directly from your GP. This is one of the friendliest customer teams in the business.

SmugglingDuds Manufacturer
Young Adults Underwear with pocket
144 Woodbine Avenue
Newcastle Upon Tyne
NE28 8HE
www.smugglingduds.com

This little known British company manufactures unique underwear products. Initially supplying the men's Smuggling Duds stash pants (boxer shorts) and the women's Smuggling Duds stash thong. They have been designed with an aesthetically pleasing pocket so you can use them to carry ("smuggle") your bag or any number of items in a unique and slick manner. These are ideal for the clubbing scene/skateboarding or just "hanging" where a bag falling from a pocket could cause extreme embarrassment.

These briefs were originally designed to carry condoms but we tested them in a nightclub scene proving their suitability to carry a spare bag that, is an ideal means of concealing a "spare" bag for emergency changes. The variety of modern colours and fabrics makes them the hottest look on the streets. Great website for ordering and now supplied with matching tee shirts and hoodies.

Surecalm Healthcare   Supplier
Ostomy supplies
Freephone: 0800854753
Email **info@surecalm.com**

Surecalm has been formed by three companies: Alphamed, BCA Direct and Homestyle Positive. All three have been established for 15 years with no bias to any appliance manufacturer!!

Friendly care team supplies product to the door. Full range of ostomy supplies.

T.G. Eakin Ltd.   Manufacturer
Ostomy & Urostomy products
15 Ballystockart Road
Comber, County Down
Northern Ireland, BT23 5QY
Telephone: **01247 871000**
www.eakin.co.uk

Unwanted Baggage

TG Eakin Limited is a medical device manufacturer, dedicated to the production of high-quality skin protection products for use in stoma and wound care. Tom Eakin, a pharmacist, formed the company in 1974. Since then, the company has gone from strength to strength and now supplies ostomy and wound care products around the world.

In 2007, TG Eakin Limited acquired **Pelican Healthcare** a leading UK supplier and manufacturer of specialist stoma and feminine health products. TG Eakin Limited is now pleased to have the opportunity to expand their international product range with Pelican Pouches. Research & Development teams within the two companies have come together to ensure the production of innovative, quality products. .

Quality is of the utmost importance at TG Eakin Limited, the company is registered as meeting the requirements of the ISO 13485:2003 standard. The staff takes great pride in producing the top-quality products and high levels of quality and hygiene are evident throughout the premises.

The company has been recognised several times for its achievements through being awarded the UK Small Business Exporter of the Year.

See **Pelican** for full range of Eakin's Products. All Eakin's products are available from all UK suppliers. Eakin's supplies its products worldwide. Its website has some excellent problem solution pages.

I can personally recommend Eakin's seals and the personal help I received in rescuing me over a weekend when all else failed, (my bag was leaking everywhere and I was desperate). An overnight package was mailed to me by Jeremy Eakin for which I am so grateful. **This is truly a personal, caring company.**

Thackraycare Supplier
Ostomy & Urostomy products
Unit 2 Landmark court
Elland Road
Leeds
LS11 8JT
Freephone: **0800 590916**
www.thackraycare.co.uk
(The website leads to Charter Healthcare)

Home delivery supplier of prescription ostomy, continence and wound care products or samples. A subsidiary of Charter Healthcare serving the Leeds area only.

UCI Healthcare Ltd Supplier
Ostomy & Urostomy products
(UCI's division Peak Medical)
Unit 8
Southill Business Park
Cornbury Park
Charlbury
Oxon
OX7 3EW
Freephone: **0800 6520420**
www.ucihealthcare.co.uk/page12.html

Unwanted Baggage

Peak Medical is UCI's distribution arm for the Netherlands range of EuroTec Ostomy products. In addition, Peak medical also caters for urostomates using Intermittent Self-Catheterisation (ISC) as a means of emptying the bladder as well as those who have undergone the Mitrofanoff Continent Diversion procedure. Samples are available on request.

<u>Vanilla Blush</u> Manufacturer
Intimate Apparel
171 Easterhill Street
Tollcross
Glasgow
G32 8LE
Telephone: 014176 30991
Email: **<u>info@vblush.com</u>**
<u>www.vblush.com</u>

Luxury Intimate apparel, swimsuits, bikinis and tankinis in a huge variety of styles to suit everyone.

They offer fantastic fabrics and lace, camis, knickers, thongs and men's boxer briefs. All designed with the discerning ostomate in mind (including the essential pouch for the bag.). New items are posted on the website at regular intervals. A refreshing change to the NHS "Bridget Jones" style ostomy knickers – **brings luxury lingerie available to ostomates!**

Victoria Health <u>Supplier</u>
<u>www.victoriahealth.com</u>

This company, featured regularly in the Mail On Sunday's You Magazine carries lines of health products that are useful to the ostomate. These include vitamin supplements, pre and post-operative supplements and essential oils some of which can help with related stoma skin problems. It is however always advisable to consult your GP or pharmacist before using any product. Victoria Health offers an online pharmacist to advise.

Weir Comfees   Manufacturer
Clothing
P.O. Box 255
Alliston, Ontario,
Canada, L9R 1V5
Telephone: **00-1- 705-434-1561** (Canada)
www.weircomfees.com/

Weir is run by a wonderful "grandmother" who started by helping an ostomy friend with her problems of finding the right underwear. She now produces a range of undergarments, bag covers and swimwear but their unique product is the:

"Comfy Drive" priced at $24.95 – It is a seat belt cover that prevents irritation to the ostomy reducing pressure from a seat belt. One size fits All! Weir is happy to export its products to the UK.

Welland Medical Ltd.   Manufacturer
Ostomy & Urostomy products
7/8 Brunel Centre
Newton Road
Crawley
West Sussex
RH10 9TU

Unwanted Baggage

Telephone: **01293 615455**
www.wellandmedical.com

Welland Medical is a British company established in 1988. It is now part of the CliniMed group of healthcare companies. It specialises in the design, development and production of stoma care pouches and accessories. Welland Medical uses the latest technology, the highest quality materials and works closely with stoma care nurses, patients and care organisations to provide innovative products to meet patient needs.

Its latest stoma product is the innovative **Flair®Active Xtra** Welland Medical's latest flushable innovation! A colostomy stoma bag for 'one-time' use in a closed format with a special adhesive so that it can be peeled off and flushed down the toilet. It is completely biodegradable.

Welland also manufacture a **unique fistula bag**. This little-known item is essential for those with fistulas surrounding the stoma. Welland products can be ordered from any supplier but its website has unique product guides which are very good, easy to follow and in video format for extra advice.

White Rose Manufacturer/Supplier
Clothing

PO Box 5121
Wimborne
Dorset
BH21 7WG

Telephone: **01202 854634**
Email: **info@whiterosecollection.com**
www.whiterosecollection.com

White Rose is a family owned and managed business, originally started due to one of the family having an ileostomy operation to create a permanent stoma after suffering with Crohn's disease. Due to this very personal involvement, the company has lots of experience of some of the problems you may encounter and have designed and chosen products that work and make things more pleasant. I have tried the sports trousers, swimsuit tankini and camis and, although I was very pleased with them all, I needed a size larger in the swimsuits than I normally wear, so check the sizing page carefully (I did not!). **A great company to deal with.**

Product range:

- Ladies Underwear and nightwear – cotton to satin in many styles
- Swimwear
- Sportswear
- Men's trousers, underwear and shorts
- Accessories including the unique "Travel john" for emptying bags in transit; Protective stoma cup for sports, travel bags and towels.

All the above companies received emails asking for their suggestive inclusions. Unfortunately, some did not reply so the information was garnered form alternative sources.

Chapter Fifteen
Benefits and Entitlements
.. Chronic Illness can bring Financial problems in its wake: Central, local government and other sources can help.

Coping with illness is a daunting task for people already exhausted by the debilitations of their illnesses, themselves. You may find that you are unable to work or that you have to leave work to care for a sick child or partner. It is understandable that you may find yourself juggling finances to make ends meet. A sensible first step is to claim the benefits to which you are entitled.

The Department of Works and Pensions - DWP's main benefit website is an excellent source of information for all those wishing to apply for benefits. They even include calculators to see if you are entitled to various means tested benefits (i.e. income support, pension credit etc.). These are strictly anonymous as you do not have to input any personal information and serve to give you a good idea whether or not you may be entitled to extra help. The website is very clear and concise, a good starting point is:

www.direct.gov.uk/en/HealthAndWellBeing/index.htm

Main applicable benefits are as follows:

DISABILITY LIVING ALLOWANCE

The government's Department of Works and Pensions (DWP) recognises that patients with chronic illnesses (i.e. Crohn's and Colitis, and/or radical surgery - bowel or bladder removal), automatically fall into the category of being able to claim Disability Living Allowance (DLA) if you are under 65.

Despite the wording, **you do not have to be physically disabled to claim this allowance**. Neither is it means tested or dependent upon your income or savings.

You may continue to receive DLA even if you return to work and you can claim DLA if you are working.

DLA comprises of three components that depend upon the amount of care you need, your general mobility and your emotional and physical state of health. Even if you are working, DLA is not included in your assessment for tax or other benefits.

Unfortunately, applying for DLA can be a nightmare. The forms are not easy to understand and claims refused on the slightest grounds. When you complete the claim pack, make sure you include supporting documentation

Unwanted Baggage

such as a letter from your GP, consultant or social services assessment team.

If you are initially declined, you must not let this put you off. Do not hesitate to go through the appeals process. It may appear daunting, but you can look forward to a lot of help with your appeals process, particularly from your county's social services department.87% of all cases submitted for appeal are accepted and the claim will be backdated to the original date of application.

To complete the initial application there are many forms of assistance.

Your local **Citizen's Advice Bureau: www.citizensadvice.org.uk**

Disability Advice Line, www.dialuk.info
If you would like to talk to a reliable, discreet resource, you can call the **Community Legal Service Helpline** on **0845 345 4 345.**

Try your local council's **Social Services Department** - you will find that they are an excellent resource.

However, for specialist knowledge relating to specific chronic illness and benefit applications, the related illness's association may also offer information to be included on your application forms. A good example is **www.crohnsandcolitis.co.uk** that provides both on-line and telephone counselling and written guides that are very easy to follow.

See: The "CROHN'S AND COLITIS UK Guide to an application for DLA" on the website.

The website will take you through the appeals process. I must stress that a very high percentage of all appeals are successful; your successful claim may be backdated to the original date of claim.

Note: The government has announced radical changes in the way that benefits are allocated. They have stated that each applicant for DLA will be expected to undergo a medical. While this can be very stressful, it is nothing to be wary of. They will examine your medical notes thoroughly and you will be given a face-to-face opportunity to state your case. **DLA does classify all ostomy patients as disabled** so the interview may not even take place. Unfortunately as things are changing it is impossible to predict the outcome at this stage. Please check with Crohn's and Colitis UK, as they seem to be the better informed of all support organisations.

Attendance Allowance

If you are over 65, then you are entitled to apply for **Attendance Allowance.** It is not means tested and does not depend upon income or savings. Similarly, the above groups will assist you with the form filling and the CROHN'S AND COLITIS UK's guide is of additional assistance:

Employment and Support Allowance This was originally known as **Incapacity benefit** but reclassified on October 2008 for applicants after that date. The old Incapacity

Unwanted Baggage

Benefit continues to be paid to claimants prior to that date.

If, due to illness, you are unable to work, the **<u>Employment and Support Allowance</u>** team offers you personalised support, advice and financial help.

It also gives you access to a specially trained personal adviser and a wide range of further services including employment, training and condition management support, to help you manage and cope with your illness or disability at work, should you wish to retrain for lighter work or carry on working under different circumstances. They will negotiate with your current employers to perhaps reduce working hours, introduce flexible working time or even allow you to work from home.

The Employment and Support Allowance involves a new medical assessment called the **Work Capability Assessment**. This assesses what you can do, rather than what you cannot, and identifies the health-related support you might need. **They do not pressure you into working in any way.** They are very sympathetic in dealing with all genuine cases.

People claiming Employment and Support Allowance may be asked to attend work focused interviews with a personal adviser. However, exclusions **are made for the chronically or long-term sick.**

Do not be intimated by the phraseology of the claim pack. **The DWP clearly do not expect you to work if you are too ill to do so. Bowel or urological surgery falls into this category**. The information pack clearly states " ***under*** *the terms of the Employment and Support Allowance, if you have an illness or disability that severely affects your ability to work, you will get increased financial support and will not be expected to prepare for a return to work".*

Be warned: Benefits and the alleged 16-hour rule

Many benefits allow the recipient to work for "16 hours" without any affect on the benefit. However, the law states, in very small print, "that a person in receipt of benefits may work **only 15.59 permitted hours per week"**.

In a recent test case brought by the DWP, a young woman had worked **one minute per week over** the actual permitted maximum for a period of eight months, – a grand total of **32** minutes. As she had exceeded the permitted work allowance time by the previously mentioned thirty-two minutes, she had to repay all the benefits she had received during this period. This was a test case brought and consequently won by the DWP, thereby setting a precedent.

Direct Payments

If you need care in your own home, you may be either eligible to receive payments from your County's social services department (Direct Payments), or the Central Government's Independent Living Fund.

Unwanted Baggage

Direct payments are monetary payments made by local councils directly to individuals who have been assessed as needing extra care services. This is particularly useful especially if you live alone and initially discharged from hospital and need help with care. Direct payments are means tested which may involve a small contribution or, awarded immediately if you are on income support or pension credit benefits.

Direct payments help people who want to manage their own support to improve their quality of life. They are designed to promote independence, choice and inclusion by enabling people to purchase the assistance or service that the council would otherwise have provided. The aim is for the patient to be fully involved in family and community life and to engage in work, education and leisure to the best of their abilities.

The government is eager to increase the number of people who receive direct payments, as such social services departments are now duty bound to consider direct payments for almost all service users who have been assessed as needing care in the home.
The direct payment system allows you to:
Have a greater input into what care you need

- Decide who you want to provide that care

- Arrange services and staff at times more convenient to your lifestyle

- Decide whether you want to employ an agency or your own staff

Your first point of contact should be your local social services team, who will send a social worker to assess your care needs.

Provided they find that you are eligible to receive help from social services, you are then entitled to ask to receive direct payments to purchase your own care rather than social services providing the care. Carers may also apply for respite help.

Eligible individuals include:

- Older and disabled people aged 16 and over, assessed as needing care.
- A person with parental responsibility for a child who is assessed as needs in care
- Carers aged 16 and over.

For further information on Direct Payments contact your local council's social services team.

After these have been awarded, you may be referred to the Rowan Organisation to help you recruit someone to help you. You do **NOT** have to use this organisation who make a large profit from administering this service. Despite guidance to the contrary from the Rowan Organisation, you can employ a family member (under certain rules – check with the council) and you can employ someone who is self-employed providing they report earnings for tax and NI purposes. If you employ someone directly then you are responsible for their NI contributions, annual leave etc.

Independent Living Fund

The Independent Living Funds were set up and funded by central government and are intended to support people with disabilities so they can live independently at home, rather than in residential care. These are intended for the severely, chronically sick.

The funds make payments to people with disabilities so they can afford to employ personal assistants or a care agency to provide the support they need to remain at home. This care may include the employment and associated employment costs of Personal Assistants or Care Agencies to help you with personal domestic tasks in your home.

There are many things that the fund cannot be used to pay for. For details, contact the fund direct on **0845 601 8815 or the** website on **www.ilf.org.uk**

To be eligible to receive payments from the fund, the person applying must:

- Be a UK resident.
- Be aged between 16 and 66.
- Receive, or have underlying entitlement to, the highest rate care component of Disability Living Allowance (DLA).
- Receive support from their Local Authority Social Services Department to the value of at least £200 per week.

- Have capital of less than £18,500.
- Expect to live at home independently for at least the next six months.

Hospital travel costs scheme

Travelling back and forth to hospitals on a regular basis can be very expensive, especially as your GP or consultant may recommend a hospital many miles away. However, you may be able to get financial help from the Hospital Travel Costs Scheme. This scheme is available if you are on a low income and need NHS treatment at a hospital, other NHS centre or private clinic and have been referred by an NHS hospital consultant.

You are automatically entitled to claim Hospital Travel Costs' Scheme, if you (or those you depend on), get at least one of the following:
- Income Support
- income-based Jobseeker's Allowance
- Income-related Employment and Support Allowance
- Guaranteed Pension Credit

You also qualify if your income is £15,050 or less and you get one of the following:

- Child Tax Credit (with or without Working Tax Credit)

Unwanted Baggage

- Working Tax Credit with the disability element or severe disability element

If an adult or your dependent child has to travel to your treatment with you for medical reasons, you can claim their travel costs too.

If you are on a low income but do not get any of these benefits or allowances, you may still claim travel costs through the NHS low income support scheme (go to section *'NHS low income support scheme'*).

If you are on entitled benefits or allowances, you will receive your full travel costs by using the cheapest form of public transport available or if you use a private car, you can claim for fuel instead (and car parking charges where unavoidable).

The hospital has a listing (which is updated regularly to reflect the changing costs of fuel), and indicates a mileage rate for fuel costs for private transport, door-to-door. It is updated to reflect fuel increases/decreases as they occur. (I checked my own car mileage with their allowance and an automobile association's guidelines for allowances and they were the same)
If you are on the NHS low-income scheme, you may get back all or some of your travel costs depending on which type of certificate you have been given.

You can claim at the **NHS hospital or clinic** at the time of your appointment. Ask for the **General Office** in the hospital, where you will receive your travel cost in cash, when you show any of the following:

- proof of a qualifying benefit (like an award notice)
- a tax credit exemption certificate (you'll get this automatically if you qualify)
- a certificate showing you qualify for the NHS low income support scheme

The NHS Low Income Support scheme

To apply for the NHS low-income support scheme, you will need to fill in form HC1.

You can order form HC1 online, by phone; call the NHS Patient Services helpline:
0845 850 1166

Your form will be assessed and, if you are entitled, you will get a certificate that confirms whether you receive full or partial help with your hospital travel costs.

If you are not able to claim at the time of a visit, keep a copy of the appointment letter and you can claim within three months of any visit (s). The hospital will give you a claim form to complete for these old appointments **NHS Planned treatment abroad /different UK regions.**

If you own health authority does not offer specific treatment to your own case, you are entitled to NHS treatment out of your own area. However, if you are referred by your consultant to another regional specialist

Unwanted Baggage

(as opposed to one within your local health board), then an application does not have to be made.

However, if you are for example, resident in Wales, and are seeking NHS treatment in a hospital based in England, then your consultant and GP may ask the Welsh Health Commission to arrange for a transfer of funding. This request normally takes about two weeks for approval to be granted. If for any reason it is declined then there is an appeals process in place. Similar applications must be processed from Scotland and Northern Ireland.

With Ostomies in mind, there is only one specialist abdominal hospital in the UK. **St Mark's** in Harrow, Middlesex handles surgical abdominal and related cases. St Mark's regularly treats residents from all UK regions, as they can offer specialist services beyond those available in Wales, Scotland and Ireland. St Marks also sees private patients without a health commission referral.

About St Mark's

www.stmarkshospital.org.uk
St. Mark's Hospital is a national and international referral centre for intestinal and colorectal disorders.
As well as clinical services covering all aspects of colorectal disease and intestinal failure, it has many research interests and a very active programme of teaching and education.

St Marks is also a large resource for publications on specifics available for download or purc*hase.*

Local Health Commissions:

In England: Primary care Trusts, practice –based commissioners and GP's deal with requests, for general information contact The Care and Quality Commission, England:

www.cqc.org.uk
In Wales: You can contact Health Commission Wales (HCW) by e-mail via hcw.enquiries@wales.gsi.gov.uk or at their address below:

Health Commission Wales (Specialist Services)
Unit 3a
Caerphilly Business Park
Caerphilly
CF83 3ED
Tel - 029 2080 7581
www.wales.gov.uk/topics/health/hcw?lang=en

?lang=en

In Scotland: You can either contact your local health board, details of which are on your medical card or from your GP or:
www.scotland.gov.uk/Topics/Health/Scrutiny
In Northern Ireland: You can contact your local health and social services boards, details of which you can obtain from your GP or contact:
www.n-i.nhs.uk

Treatment Abroad on the NHS

If you are thinking of going to another country specifically for medical treatment, different rules apply than those for getting necessary care whilst abroad on a trip. It is important to note that your European Health Insurance Card (EHIC) does **not** cover going abroad for planned treatment. Have a look ay the NHS website:

http://www.nhs.uk/nhsengland/Healthcareabroad/pages/healthcareabroad.aspx

First, you should discuss your plans with your GP or consultant **before you make any travel or make medical arrangements.** They will refer you to your local health commissioner who will discuss the options available to you and will confirm the following:

- Which treatments they are prepared to fund, and what level of funding would be available.

- Exactly how much you will be reimbursed.

- That you fully understand the conditions under which you will be treated abroad.

- Any programme of after-care or follow-up treatment you might require upon your return to the UK.

If going to an EU country, there are two routes for obtaining NHS funding. You can use the E112 form issued by the Overseas Healthcare Team (Newcastle) or, alternatively, you can go under Article 49 of the EC treaty. Your local commissioner can advise you on which option is better for the type of treatment you require. Each option works in a slightly different way. This availability of treatment is used much more often than you might think and is a serious alternative to areas with a long NHS waiting list.

Utility Benefits:

Water and Sewerage Charges.
To meter or not?

You cannot switch your water provider, as, while the market is privatised, it is not open to competition and are limited to the company that owns the water provision within your region. This means your most important decision is how you are billed.

Water Bills – the traditional way

Only 30% of homes have a water meter, most are still being charged on the 'water bill' system. Here the price is fixed depending on a home's 'rateable value', and the amount of water used is irrelevant.

This means that the more your home can be rented out for, the more you will pay. It is staggering that even though rates were abolished in 1990, water bills still depend on them. There are no plans to change this archaic system and, unfortunately, no prospect of getting your home's value re-assessed (unless the water company decides to re-assess your whole area).

The average un-metered bill in England and Wales is a whopping £362, while the average metered bill is £309

Unwanted Baggage

– though it varies heavily with region. However, while in England and Wales (though not Scotland or Northern Ireland), water companies are privatised, there is still no competition. You cannot switch to a different water company – as you can in the gas and electricity markets - to get a cheaper supplier

It is important first to see whether a meter is financially worthwhile. As a rough rule of thumb, if there are more bedrooms in your house than people, you should investigate getting a meter

Whether a water meter is worthwhile depends on your Water Company and usage. This calculation can be done two ways for you:

For a quick calculation, both comparison sites Uswitch and the Consumer Council for Water offer calculators:
www.uswitch.com/water
www.ccwater.org.uk/server.php?show=nav.388

The Uswitch one is much easier to use, it questions how often you use the washing machine and dishwasher and the number of showers and baths taken weekly by your household. This can often be more than you think. Four people showering daily = 28 showers a week. Once details have been input, it quickly calculates whether a meter will cut your bills in most areas of England and Wales.

Alternately, you can ask your water Company do conduct an assessment for you.

Water - Benefit/Illness reductions

If you have a water meter and someone in your household receives benefits it may be possible to get the amount you pay capped. To be eligible you need to be receiving benefits or have three or more children under the age of 19. Alternatively, if someone in your household has a medical condition that means they use a lot of extra water, you are also entitled to a capped fee. **All ostomates qualify under these qualifications**

If you are accepted your costs will be limited to the average household bill for your water company however much water you use. Average savings can be around £250/year. To sign up contact your water board for an application. The application must be made before the beginning of the water board's official year (April) to be effective for the following year.

If you are on private sewerage (septic tank), they will still cap your water rate.

Electric and Gas Charges

If you are in receipt of any benefits, Or, in cases of medical use of electric, all the gas or electric companies will apply a reduction to your bill. In most cases, this reduction will be applied from the date of your telephone call.

For further details of special rates and emergency supply arrangements for the chronically sick contact your suppliers on their customer service numbers.

Unwanted Baggage

If you have difficulty in paying your bills and are worried about being cut off, contact your county's social services department who will liaise on your behalf with the utility companies concerned.

Telephone

Most telephone companies buy or rent lines or time from BT. As such they do not offer any discounts or make any provision to those who are disabled or chronically sick as their rates are already discounted.

BT itself offers special discounts and help to people on benefits or to those who are chronically sick. . There are a number of different schemes including BT Basic,

BT Basic

If you are in receipt of benefits, and are a BT subscriber for incoming calls, then you are entitled to the BT Basic rate. The BT Basic line rental is only £13.20 every quarter. Your line rental includes a call allowance of £4.50 every three months. This means that if your phone calls to normal UK or international destinations never go over that amount, your bill will never be more than £13.20. For an application form, telephone:
0800 783 1675

BT's Protected Service

Unfortunately, BT has to disconnect phone lines when the phone bill has not been paid. There may be a good reason for this, for example you may have had a sudden stay in hospital, or you might sometimes find it difficult manage your day-to-day affairs. BT's Protected Service scheme lets you choose someone you trust to act on your behalf. This could be a friend, a relative or someone such as a social worker who agrees to be your representative. Social services are excellent at handling this service on your behalf and may offer financial aid in settling an outstanding bill.

If your telephone bill is not paid on time, BT will contact your chosen person by telephone or letter to help BT sort out the problem. There is no charge for this service and your chosen person will not have to pay the bill out of his or her own money. BT is aware of the difficulties of how ill health can affect a person's financial position, through this scheme; they will negotiate a regular payment and ensure the telephone stays connected. For more information, call BT customer service on:

0800 800 150

BT Repairs

Free Priority Fault Repair scheme
The telephone is a vital lifeline for people who are unable to leave the house because of an illness or disability. If you have a chronic long-term illness or a severe disability, you can apply for BT's Free **Priority Fault Repair Scheme.** BT does ask for your application to be supported by a medical practitioner. Once you are registered, BT will deal with reported faults as soon as possible, day or night, 365 days a year. To get an application form, please call:

Unwanted Baggage

0800 800 151

Other financial Help for telephone bills: If you are having difficulty affording to pay for your BT phone service, there are a number of organisations and charities that may be able to help:

For those over 60, Age Concern provides a free fact sheet called "Help with Telephones". For further details, telephone Age Concern or visit the websites.
For England: **www.ageconcern.or.uk**
Age Concern Scotland, telephone: 0845 125 9732 (local call rates) Monday to Friday, 10am – 4pm**. The** website is:
www.olderpeoplescotland.co.uk

Age Concern Cymru, Units 13 & 14 Neptune Court, Vanguard Way, Cardiff CF24 5PJ, telephone: 029 2043 1555 (national call rate); website:
www.accymru.org.uk

Age Concern Northern Ireland, 3 Lower Crescent, Belfast BT7 1NR, telephone: 028 9032 5055 (national call rate) Monday to Friday 10.00am - 12pm and 2pm – 4pm, website:
www.ageconcernni.org

Communicability

This charity was set up in the memory of former BT employee, James Powell.

This trust helps with the provision of communications aids, equipment and related services to disabled people. For further details, visit the Communicability website **www.communicability.smartchange.org**

Television

Caught in the digital switchover?
Help is at hand - BBC's **Switchcover Help Scheme** is available to anyone at a small charge, or **FREE** to all those on pension credits, income support, attendance allowance, disability allowance or jobseeker's allowance or those aged 75 or over.

This service will help people in these categories to convert one of their TV sets to digital.

They will install easy-to-use equipment that meets your need and fit the necessary dish, if it is needed to make the new equipment work. You must also have a valid TV licence. It also includes 12 months aftercare.
Call free on **0800 4085900** for more information or visit **www.helpscheme.co.uk**

Extra Funds available for all needs

Family Action's Welfare Grants
http://www.family-action.org.uk/section.aspx?id=8301

Telephone: **020 7254 6251**
Family Action's Welfare Grants are available for clothing and general household needs such as beds and cookers

but they can also help with more varied needs such as communication aids and medical adaptations. While there are no set limits, in general grants are made for £100 to £300. If you need a larger grant, you should also explore funding from other sources or revise the amount you are seeking, before submitting an application. You might find it helpful to search for other sources of funding at Turn2us

By visiting their website, you will be able to carry out a search of grant-giving charities.

Who can receive a grant?

Welfare Grants mainly assist families and individuals with low incomes, particularly those living on benefits. Grants are available to people from across the UK. These grants are for the benefit of the whole family, for example, they would consider might a grant for appliances such as a new washing machine.

Welfare Grant applicants must fall into one or more of the following priority areas to be eligible for funding.

Priority Areas

- **Mental Health**: (over the age of 18) support to improve the quality of life and reduce isolation for families or individuals with mental health problems.

- **Domestic abuse**: support for those leaving a violent relationship to help rebuild their lives.

- **Refugees and asylum seekers**: support to promote the stability of families and individuals and their integration into life in the UK.

- **Older people**: Support to promote independence, improve the quality of life and reduce isolation for those aged 60 and over.

- **Young people (aged 19 to 25)**: Support for vulnerable young people to help to establish a stable and independent life.

- **Sickness/disability**: Small grants for medical treatment (particularly special treatment), services, facilities or equipment for those who are sick or physically disabled.

Turn2us

Financial assistance and other forms of support are often available from grant-giving organisations, depending on particular background and circumstances.

This fantastic website contains a database of over 3000 funds offering welfare grants. An assisted search applies a step-by-step wizard to collect details of your background, occupation and location to find the best match between your needs and funds that might be able to help.

www.turn2us.org.uk/grants_search/search_by_topic.aspx

Chapter Sixteen
Emotions
Emotional adjustment to life with a chronic Illness

After undergoing any serious surgery, all patients find that their emotional state has changed together with any physical changes that surgery may have caused. When we are healthy, we tend to think of our bodies as somehow intact. Major surgery can shatter that image, and with it the concept of self-satisfying health. The feelings of loss and vulnerability can be profound, and recognizing depression in any surgery's aftermath becomes very important.

In particular, it is difficult to describe the pain that bowel or urinary illnesses can cause. Most ostomy patients will have suffered excruciating pain for a year or more before surgery. It is inevitable that this intense pain will have caused you to experience a gamut of emotions. Painkillers unfortunately only served to take the edge of this kind of pain. You may have been left feeling frustrated, tired, debilitated, angry and afraid. You will have slept to avoid the pain or suffered from insomnia, waking frequently as pain increases. There comes a time when you will do anything to be relieved of this pain – an operation and a stoma seems the only logical conclusion.

Bowel surgery involves major extensive emotional and physical scarring. You will still experience a degree of discomfort for some time after your operation. Initially you will still tire easily and may not be able to return to "normal", as soon as you hoped. Physically your stoma will appear very red and swollen. The discharge is smelly and your bag experiences may be difficult at first with potential leakage and skin problems. The swelling will recede. Odour can easily be controlled by the bag filter and added in-bag deodorants. Your skin will adjust. Your physical scars will heal, although some permanent scarring is inevitable. Changing and emptying the bag will become routine. Physical life will become manageable.

However, it is important for you to understand that your emotional reactions after surgery can be very intense. This is because the operation has changed your body. These changes are both sudden and significant. The fact that you can no longer control faecal output represents an acute loss of bodily function. Emotionally you may feel shocked and tense; you may also feel disgust about your stoma. You may assume that others will think the same way about you. In reality, they will be relieved that you are out of pain. The bag will feel awkward; you may believe that everyone will notice the bump under your clothes when it is relatively inconspicuous to others. You may be worried about your future health and ongoing medical care.

It is important to recognise that these worries can make you feel weepy, sad and depressed. This is normal. You must share these feelings with those closest to you and may be surprised to find that they are feeling the same way on your behalf. Thy will be angry that you have had to

Unwanted Baggage

endure the pain of surgery and the obvious changes that have happened to you through no fault of your own. They may be frustrated that they cannot help as much as they would like to. As long as you and your family, carers and close friends are open and honest with each other about your feelings, you can move on and begin to see life anew with even a little humour on the vagaries of your stoma and its bag.

If your operation was an emergency procedure, you will not have had time to prepare yourself for the adjustments involved with bodily changes. This can cause a much more serious depression – it is essential that you confide your deepest fears to those closest to you, so that they can reassure you that they accept and love you for who you are.

Getting through the first six months can be a challenge. You will have to make difficult adjustments but you will soon be able to enjoy such things as mild exercise, sex and the simple joy of eating again. Keep expressing your feelings no matter how difficult it may seem, as this will help you.

You may also think that you have made a good emotional adjustment. However, in some cases, postoperative depression can occur well after the crisis of surgery has ended and you have been at home for some time. This sudden onset of depression can make it much more difficult for patients to cope with feelings about what they have endured and what their future is likely to be, or for family members and caregivers, to see and understand their feelings, especially as you may have presented an initial cheerful face to the world. If this happens, try to explain how you feel and how the realisation of what has happened has finally dawned on you. The more you can talk about your emotional rollercoaster, the better you will feel.

In the final analysis, you have a choice - you can either present yourself to the world as a sick person or a well person. If you choose the role of a sick person, you will give people the impression that the only thing that matters about you is your stoma and any other illness that you may have. If you do this, you will be treated as an invalid.

On the other hand you can be as well as you can, treating the stoma as incidental and trying to do as much as you can to live life to the full – I will not use the word "normal" – there is no such thing as normality – but you have to roll with the punches. Life is not fair; yes, you have a stoma and may suffer from other associated illnesses, flare-ups, and post-operative complications that you must deal with. If you are positive, people will then continue to involve you in their lives and activities. Your alternatives are to become bedbound and even isolated. Self-pity is self-destructive. That is no way to live life or to share your life with friends and family. Take those days that you do not feel a hundred percent and indulge yourself with a little bed rest. Treat yourself to special foods that you may fancy, read a book, watch a film - enjoy yourself and others will enjoy you and your company.

If you do find that, after an initial period of adjustment, you still have difficulty in coping with all the changes that have taken place, seek professional help. A patient who is enlightened enough to want to explore this route will help

Unwanted Baggage

to speed the mental healing process. Initially, you should contact your GP who will refer to you the appropriate consultant. Many local health boards are taking an innovative approach to post operative depression; help may not involve medication, there are many other routes available including cognitive behaviour therapy and group counselling and even yoga.

If for any reason you do not wish to consult your GP in the first instance, there is an excellent website
Depression Alliance for **England** (only):
www.depressionalliance.org
Telephone: **08451232320**
Depression Alliance has counselling groups throughout England and offers many self-help guides.

Depression Alliance Scotland is:
www.dascot.org
Telephone**: 0845 1232320**

Community Advice and Listening Line (CAL):
This is unique to **Welsh NHS** patients but is a good starting point for seeking further help and advice. It operates a helpline service on:
Telephone: **0800 132 737**

An independent advice service for depression in **Wales** supports a network of self-help groups throughout Wales is **Journeys OnLine.**
Telephone: **029 2069 2891**
www.journeysonline.org.uk

Aware Defeat Depression supports all those affected in **Northern Ireland.** They also welcome enquiries

Elizabeth Prosser & Philip Prosser

from support workers, family and carers. They have an established network of twenty support groups throughout the country.

www.aware-ni.org
Telephone: **08451 202961**

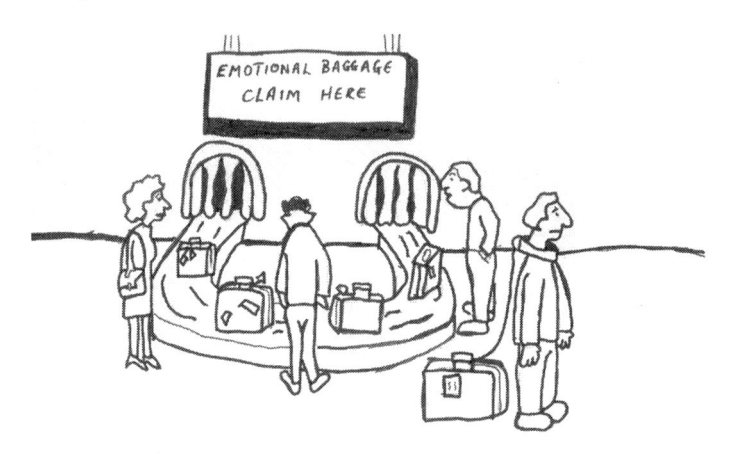

Chapter Seventeen
Intimacy
.. Up close and personal

Intimacy is part of any relationship between two consenting adults. Intimacy includes tenderness, touching and kissing. These are all part of lovemaking. Lovemaking includes sex that is the most intimate act that two human beings can engage in. We are all sexual beings. Young, old, male, female, heterosexual, gay, or whether or not we have a stoma –Engaging in lovemaking is a natural, important, pleasurable experience.

However, lying in a hospital bed looking down at your new stoma and its attached bag you may not be thinking too much about making love! Long standing spouses or partners will have accompanied you during the traumatic experience of your illness and surgery. If you ask that your partner be present in the hospital on an occasion when your bag is changed, then, there will be no surprises when returning home, you take your clothes off and share a bed.

For a couple in a loving, caring relationship, this is just a new learning curve. Naturally, your partner will be concerned and they may wish to talk to the surgeon or stoma nurse alone to be reassured that, for an ostomist, sex can be as usual it was before surgery.

Recovery and adjustment from any major surgery takes time. There are no set guidelines as to when you can resume sex – it will be when you feel comfortable, both mentally and physically.

Logistics

Essentially, there are a few points to address. You now have a bag and some scarring. If you are initially uncomfortable naked, women might be more at ease during sex if they wear a "boob tube", belly band or chemise top to hide the bag or any scarring. If you wear a transparent bag, a good idea is to wear a discreet bag cover – they come in attractive colours and patterns. (See the accessories section for manufacturers or instructions on how to make one). There is one available in a velvet heart shape! Men may prefer to tape the bag to the skin to hold it in position or, again wear a bag cover. White Rose (see accessories), makes special crotch-less silk underwear that will hold the bag firmly in place, while disguising the bag.

It is of course necessary to empty your bag before making love, as additional pressure on a full or half-empty bag may cause the bag to come detached or burst. You can also wear a smaller bag, especially designed for bathing or lovemaking i.e. the DANSAC mini 22920.

One important point about wearing a small bag is that during orgasm, the stoma may spasm, filling the bag. One way of preventing this is not to eat for at least four hours before making love. This involves a certain lack of spontaneity but is, unfortunately, necessary.

Unwanted Baggage

The big question – How do ostomists make love? The BIG answer is the same way as people so without stomas! In saying that, I must make it clear that the bag does get in the way and does impede easy athletic movements, but trying adjustments in position can help. You may not be the acrobat you once were and initially there will be some awkwardness as you adjust to positions that are more comfortable.

Think back to the time you first met - the time when you first made love. This was a time that you took to find out about each other exploring and discovering new things. It is just like that, a new exciting beginning.

The most important thing is communication and a sense of humour. You must tell each other if anything is painful or if you feel embarrassed in any way. Your partner may be afraid of hurting you, which may in turn affect his or her reactions. Do not give up at the first hurdle. Begin with some gentle holding, kissing and tenderness and let nature take its course.

Patience is also an issue. A man, after a period of abstinence may be overexcited which can lead to a temporary situation of premature ejaculation. In some instances temporary impotence could occur, not because your partner sees you as unattractive but simply out of fear of hurting you (as the ostomist) or himself (as the ostomist), or damaging the stoma in some way. It all takes time and perhaps a few glasses of your favourite tipple! If this situation continues, then do consult your stoma nurse or your GP who will be happy to offer further guidance.

If an ostomist acquires a new, potential sexual partner, it is wise to explain that you have an appliance. You should explain that you have had a non-contagious, serious illness that had to be treated surgically. The result is that you now wear a permanent bag. This should be done before you feel too attached to someone, so think about telling your story, even on a first date, then no one can say you did not prepare them properly. You might like to carry some literature about your illness with you so that they fully understand.

You must realise that if you whisper this tenderly in your partner's ear in a moment of extreme passion, this one surprise may make the situation intolerable for you both.

Plan, by rehearsing a short explanation to yourself; once you have decided how to talk about your situation, it will be easier to find time to explain to a potential new partner.

It is important to give a prospective partner time to consider the situation. Beginning a physical relationship too soon, without proper communication may end in disaster. A prospective partner may reject you at some point. However, this rejection may not be a result of the stoma at all . In any event, if someone does not want you with a stoma, it is unlikely that a meaningful relationship would have prospered.

Unwanted Baggage

"I'm not usually fond of blind dates but I think tonight went well!"

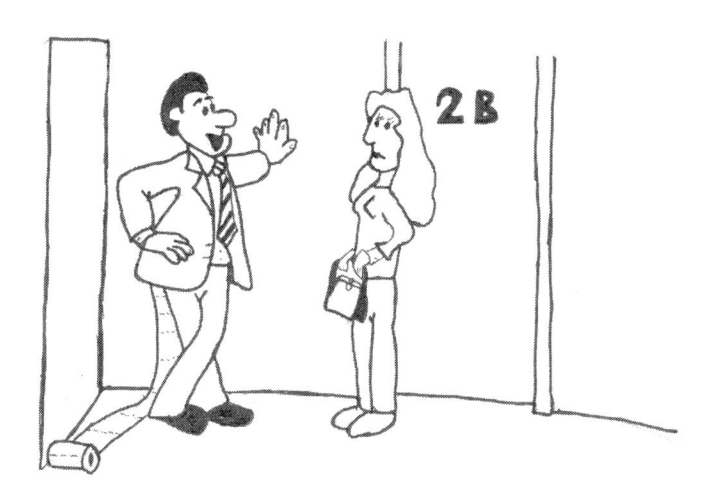

Casual Sex

In today's modern world, casual sex is common. Unfortunately, for the ostomist this does not always result in a pleasurable encounter. There have been instances where ostomists have relied on taping over the stoma as a quick method of disguising the situation. This will not work. The stoma cannot be relied on. When you least expect it, it may gush forth taking the tape with it, embarrassing everyone. Starving yourself for hours, in the hope of draining the stomal duct will not work either. This could cause a long-term negative effect upon your health, as it is very important to eat regularly. Wearing a "belly band" or the specially designed crotchless underwear will disguise the bag and hold it in place. A small bag, such as the Dansac mini, can also be used providing you carry a spare with you at all times.

Contraception

If you have been using the Pill as a contraceptive, do check with your GP, as there is evidence that the contraceptive affect of the pill may pass through into the bag without being absorbed into the body. In these circumstances, the protection of the pill is lost. Other methods of contraception are not affected. Good alternatives are the coil, condom or patch.

Specifics for the male ostomist

The greatest difficulties that men are likely to encounter post-operatively are erectile problems. This highly complex phenomenon may occur in men of all ages, and can occur for many reasons that have nothing to do with surgery directly. It is obviously not a problem unique to stoma patients.

Sometimes this occurs because the man believes or comes to believe that he will be unable to have an erection or climax. It then becomes a cycle of failure, loss of belief and continued failure.

The process is usually made worse by the fact that the failure in the act of making love causes tension between partners. The woman may not feel frustrated, but may feel that her lover no longer finds her attractive and that is why he cannot or will not make love to her. She feels

Unwanted Baggage

rejected and the whole relationship takes a downwards turn. The biggest sex organ is the brain, if you believe you cannot – you will not.

Sometimes some simple changes can help. A warm relaxing bath before bedtime, plenty of rest and adequate diet all contribute. Lack of pressure or stress is very important. There are many ways to please your partner other than intercourse. Alternatively, try kissing, cuddling, caressing your partner, do everything but attempt intercourse. After a few sessions of foreplay alone, intercourse may follow easily. If you can achieve an erection through masturbation or wake up with an erection, you are certainly not impotent.

In some cases, the causes of impotence following stoma surgery are genuinely physical. For male stoma patients there is a risk that the nerves governing erection and ejaculation may be damaged during surgery. Erection comes about because of stimuli travelling along the parasympathetic nerve pathways. These fibres run close to the rectum. If these fibres are damaged in surgery, the ability to have an erection will be wholly or partially lost. Ejaculation is dependent on the sympathetic nervous system. These pathways are vulnerable in surgery too. Impotence is more usual for men having a colostomy than an ileostomy because there is less damage to the tissues in the latter and therefore less risk to the nerve pathways.

Surgery for bowel cancer is extensive and therefore more damaging. According to the available data on this topic, age seems to be an important factor, with older men having more problems. Whether the cause is that older men are more likely to have a colostomy than ileostomy (because bowel cancer is more common in older age groups), is far from clear. Temporary impotence is not unusual following stoma surgery, or surgery of any kind, so do not think that all is lost if, within a couple of months after surgery, you have not begun to have sexual relations. The healing process sometimes takes a long time.

Even in the ultimate case of permanent impotence, there are solutions. Over the last few years, medical science has developed surgical techniques that can help some impotent men, including ostomists. This type of surgery is highly specialised. In the first instance, you should talk to your colorectal surgeon or your GP about this kind of approach.

If the impotence is not physical but continues after the first three months following surgery, seek advice from your GP, who may then prescribe Viagra or arrange specialised counselling.

A comfortable position is important. Again, look on this as an opportunity to explore new positions that do not put undue pressure on the bag. Taping the bag in place is an excellent idea and a good bag cover will disguise it.

Specifics for the female ostomist

Having a stoma is not a bar to intercourse or having children. Normal birth with normal vaginal delivery is quite feasible. This is dependent on the reproductive organs being undamaged and working normally.

As far as the mechanics of sexual intercourse are concerned, there are several, typical problems that the female stoma patient might experience.

- If the rectum is removed, then problems may relate to the way the perineal wound heals. (The wound left when the rectum is removed). It sometimes remains tender for a considerable time following surgery and thus sexual intercourse can be painful.

- Sometimes, the space left when the colon is removed allows the uterus to shift backwards. This can cause pain during intercourse.

- Some female ostomists may find that there is a decrease in feeling and sensitivity of the clitoris. This may be because the nerve pathways to the clitoris are impaired during surgery.

- A frequent problem is vaginal dryness that makes intercourse difficult and uncomfortable.

- Penetration may be painful and uncomfortable, simply because of the scarring of the tissues following removal of the colon or bladder.

There are a number of solutions. For dryness, a lubricating jelly, cream or pessaries can be applied in advance. If your partner wears a condom, which is lubricated, this may also help. If the perineal wound continues to be a problem, then surgical reconstruction of the perineal wound, particularly if sinuses are present, can help enormously.

If penetration is painful, then you should try altering positions – a good variation is then spooning or the scissor position may be more comfortable. If the rectum has been removed, the missionary position (the female laying on her back with her partner on top of her) may be initially uncomfortable. One solution is for the man to enter the vagina from behind, the female kneeling with her knees apart with the man kneeling behind. The other alternative is for the woman to sit astride her partner who lays on his back while she guides his penis into her vagina.

Timing and communication are very important. Do not try to have intercourse too soon after surgery. – A good medium is about six weeks after you have been discharged from hospital. If you feel well enough before then, go ahead. Do not be afraid to say "no". Your considerate partner will understand but do not make him feel rejected. Explain that it is not him, that although you feel aroused, intercourse is causing you discomfort.

There are other ways to please your partner. You can explore the world of sexual toys and mutual masturbation and oral sex. Sometimes, if undue pressure seems to be the problem than accessories, such as a specialised swing or frame that takes the weight, may be the answer.

Heterosexual Anal sex

If surgery has been carried out on the bowel, the rectum may have been removed and a rectal stump may be left. This is not usually enough to allow anal sex. If it is attempted, can result in extreme pain, bleeding and damage requiring surgery or total rectum removal. If in doubt, ask your GP or consultant.

Homosexuality

For homosexual men and lesbian women, having a stoma is not in itself any more or less of a problem than for heterosexuals.

Other things being equal, a homosexual man will be able to have an erection and ejaculate. The big problem facing a man is, if he has used his rectum as a receptive sex organ. The rectum may be removed in surgery, although this depends upon the operative procedure and the type and extent of the disease and consequent risk to the life of the patient.

Given that the decision to remove the rectum is to some extent a matter of clinical judgment, it is important for a gay man to discuss the issue with the surgeon pre-operatively to explore the possibility of keeping as much of the rectum in place and any risks that might arise from doing so. It is usually possible for a surgeon to reconstruct the rectum so that it can be used sexually. It is important however, that you verify this before and after surgery to ensure that anal sex is now possible.

A suitable period of healing (usually three months), must be allowed and you should check with your GP or stoma nurse as to when sexual relations can be resumed. If there is any pain or bleeding, you must immediately seek medical advice.

In cases where the rectum has to be removed, the stoma must not be used in any way as a substitute. **Serious, possibly fatal damage** can be caused by inserting anything into the stoma other than by a medical professional's examination.

Lesbian women usually prove to be empathetic ostomy partners. They have a better understanding on how the female body works and therefore can sometimes adjust more easily to being an ostomist or ostomist's partner than those in a heterosexual relationship. Again positioning, time and communication is all important to comfortable sex.

General Advice

Tiredness, Fatigue

Many people recovering from ostomical surgery may feel "washed out" and almost without energy for several weeks after surgery. It is not unusual for this to last for many months. This lethargy can make people lose interest in sex. In most cases, counselling alone may help, medication to enhance mood or simply vitamin supplements may help.

HRT is also available, (hormone replacement therapy), this can replace testosterone in both men and women which, in turn, will increase libido. It can be given as tablets, injections or patches.

Talk to your GP or stoma nurse in the first instance and they will advise on the best treatment or counselling that you may need.

Body Image

After any surgery, you may feel depressed. Part of this depression can be the change in how we *think* our body has been affected by surgery. In turn this can affect your self-confidence. We also have strong mental attachments to our bodies and when a change occurs this can cause emotional damage as well as surgical changes. The surgical changes have removed, to an extent the privacy of your bowel functions. Now, you wear a bag on your side that contains faecal or urinary discharge. The bag will not go away. It cannot be surgically disguised or reconstructed. Your mind has to make a terrific adjustment to allow acceptance of what is essentially a new body part. If you cannot accept it, you will imagine that no one else can or, to that end, cannot love you. Logically you know that this is not true. However, logic does not always play a part in how we feel or how we think others feel.

It is very important to talk about how you feel and encourage your partner to discuss his or her feelings with you. You may think they are disgusted by this change – it is essential to bring these feelings out in the open so that you can both relax and learn to love the new "you".

Most partners will be delighted to know that you are out of the pain that caused the operation. In time, you and your partner will learn to make the necessary mental adjustments to return to a complete sexual relationship.

Communication is the key issue that will help solve underlying sexual problems after surgery. Never be afraid to say "no" if you are in pain, tired or feeling lethargic – if you go through the motions, your partner will sense that your heart is not in it and may feel rejected. It is far better to say "no", explain why and enjoy a comforting cuddle. If a position is painful, say so. Pain is a warning that something is not right. Listen to your body, and change to a more comfortable position, explain why and have fun experimenting! Re-read "The joy of sex" and giggle over the "Kama Sutra"!

Counselling Resources

If you are seriously depressed, you must seek professional medical advice. Initially talk to our GP or stoma nurse. If you think that you are not getting enough help or understanding, then find a good psychosexual counsellor.

- The Institute of Psychosexual Medicine **www.ipm.org.uk**

- The British Sexual and Relationship Therapy Organisation can advise on counsellors in your area. If there is a serious sexual dysfunction issue through surgery **www.bast.org.uk**

- The Sexual Dysfunction Association has many fact sheets for both men and women to offer advice and solutions and the website has contacts for further help. **www.sda.org.uk**

Sex for all can be fun and is a very important part of life. If you have initial problems after the operation, do persevere, there will be a solution.

Chapter Eighteen
Children and Young People
... the world of young ostomates

If you are a parent of a child with an ostomy, you will have many questions and concerns. Your specialist will have assured you that the ostomy surgery was necessary. This however does not preclude feelings of shock, fear or even guilt. Initially, your doctor and stoma nurse will do all they can to help you deal with the emotions that you will have. Your consultant, GP, stoma nurse will all help you attend to your child's physical needs. It is at times like these it is important to share your feelings with family and friends and you may choose to seek professional counselling for both yourself and your young ostomist.

The age at which the ostomical surgery is performed has a strong bearing on the kind of support he or she will need. From the outset, you should involve your child at all medical appointments, if your child is three or older, encourage the doctor to talk your child directly, as well as addressing you, the parents. He or she is the patient! Research shows that children who feel that you are involving them and take their involvement seriously, helps them to deal with difficult situations more easily than those whose views are taken for granted (ref: Ruth Sinclair "Involving children in their care" 1998). As a parent, you should:

- Provide information so that children and young people can contribute meaningfully to any decisions regarding their healthcare management.

- Give your child both the time and the relevant explanations so that they can properly understand the issues and the process involved in any planned procedures, tests and operations.

- Be clear about what will happen, and the likely consequences.

- As soon as your child is computer literate, encourage them to access information about their illness on the internet and through the various children's' forums and websites – Medikiz is good! (See below for details).

- Make sure that both you and your child is comfortable talking to their assigned health professionals – the consultant, the surgeon, the GP and the stoma nurse who will all play a very important part in your child's life. Address any concerns they may have and discuss any problems with the relevant person.

If your child is three or older, then pre-operative play is important. You can play at "operations" and practice sticking a bag on and off each other and teddy as well! (Your stoma nurse will be glad to provide you with samples).

One of the most difficult things about being a young person with any chronic condition is the isolation that comes about with being different. The simple stoma emerges as a problem when the child begins nursery or school. It is essential to discuss with the teaching staff, the help that your child may need and to warn them of possible problems, such as bag leakages etc. You may wish to put together a kit for the teacher to keep in a safe place as well as a change of clothing. While teachers are used to dealing with "accidents" in the classroom, they may not have encountered a "bag" and it is important for them to realise that your child can lead a normal life but may need help on occasion.

On the subject of teasing and bullying, children are usually brutally honest. They will discover anything that makes a classmate somehow different (glasses, hearing aids, diabetics or even different colour hair), and they may make fun of them. Anything that makes children feel that one of them is different worries them, as they may be unable to understand the reasons. There is no fast or easy answer to this. You can ask the teachers to explain to the class, using a condition specific doll.

These dolls are made for a number of illnesses and are used as teaching tools to form a psychological bridge to help other children understand. An ostomy doll can be customised in skin shades, male of female sex, complete with a small ostomy bag that can be removed to show a stoma underneath. Although they can act as a teaching aid, they are also great "pals" who have an ostomy too! – These wonderful dolls even come in adult and granny versions to amuse the older ostomate!

You should realise that even young children are more aware than you may think and they need your respect and trust in helping them deal with their condition.

The Cleveland Clinic Foundation in Ohio is the only resource that has actively studied the effects of ostomy surgery performed on children between the ages of six and twelve years of age with regard to their psychological development during childhood and subsequent development during adolescence.

Out of the subjects studied, seven out of ten adjusted well in the first years after surgery. Key factors in good adjustment were support from the family and a perception of normalcy, specifically including the management of their own ostomy care. However, all subjects reported that the ostomy had a negative impact on their lives during adolescence.

Ostomate Teens that had contact with each other during their key stage of development fared much better than those who did not. The age at which the subjects originally underwent ostomical surgery did not influence the difficulties reported during adolescence. In conclusion, the report stated categorically that ostomical surgery performed on children can have long-term psychosocial effects on adolescent development. The key answer in addressing these effects was education about ostomy care for themselves, paramount at the early stages, followed by referral to mutual support groups for both parents and children through the adolescent phase.

Communication – talking to your young person - is paramount. Do not guess what they are thinking – ask them, involve them in discussions with the specialist and GP - even a young child will understand more than you think.

Most of all encourage them to ask the medical team questions or discuss with them any worries they may have. The varying stomas may bring separate problems but you should discuss these with your child at all times.

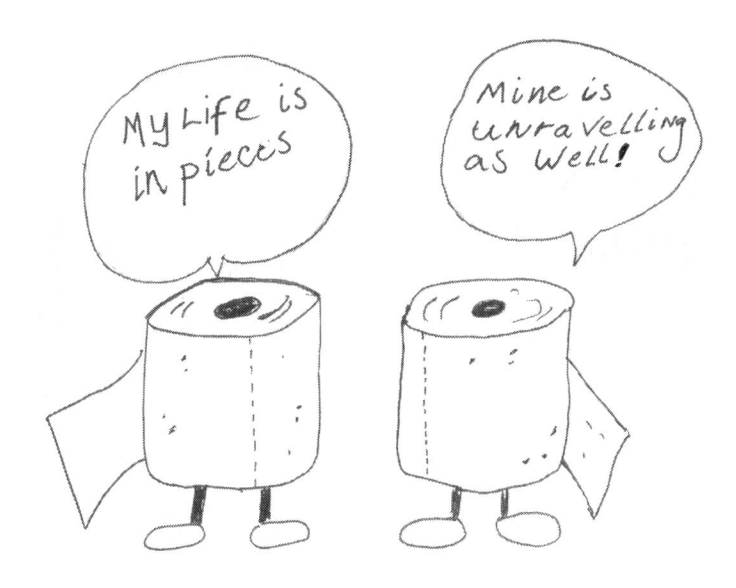

> My Life is in pieces

> Mine is unravelling as well!

Siblings – If your baby has brothers or sisters, it is essential that you talk about baby's ostomy as soon as possible, let them see you changing baby and let them look at the stoma. You should explain that your new baby is not sick but has to wear a bag instead of going to the toilet the usual way. They might like to help by fetching supplies and keeping baby amused while you change the bag. As with any new arrival in the family, it is essential that they not feel neglected or left out. For younger siblings, a present of an ostomy doll will let them change their doll's bag while you change baby's.

Baby and Toddler Ostomates

A number of babies are born with bowel and bladder problems needing an ostomy at birth or soon after. The hospital will show you how to clean the stoma, empty the bag and apply new ones. They will make sure you are comfortable with the changing procedure before baby leaves hospital. The same system applies for babies as it does for adults although you may seek to find milder cleansing agents or creams. Again, the hospital and stoma nurse will advise you. Your stoma nurse will visit regularly as baby grows and you can rely on her for help and assistance on specialist bags, as they are needed. He or she will monitor the skin around the stoma and advise on treatment if it becomes irritated.

Most bag manufacturers supply baby and toddler sized bags. These usually come with attractive animal designs but a bag cover is strongly recommended to prevent rubbing. **Bullens** make soft cotton covers in attractive designs and will make covers from your own material. All covers are made-to-measure per specific bag.

Ideally, change the bag either early in the morning before the first feed or at bath-time before a last feed. It is usually more convenient to empty the bag with nappy changes. You may find you can empty the bag onto the soiled nappy. If you find this impractical, a small disposable kidney dish can be used (placed strategically!). One bag should last for twenty-four hours.

You may bathe baby with or without the bag – water will not affect the stoma, but check with your doctor if your baby has a urostomy bag, as he may not wish this kind of stoma to be covered in water. Avoid using oil or oily soaps in the water as this may prevent the new bag from sticking properly. Do not use baby oil or powder on the skin surrounding the stoma for the same reason. If baby is bathed with the bag on, remove it as quickly as possible. A wet bag will soon irritate the skin surrounding it.

You can take baby swimming but ensure that a bag is in place at all times.

As a child becomes more active, crawling and walking, the stoma will become more active – check the bag periodically to stop it from bursting.

Clothing is also very important. As a baby or toddler grows, they begin to dress and undress themselves, this is the time when they pull at the bag or try to dislodge it. They may be uncomfortable in clothing with stiff or buttoned/zippered waistbands. Some basic guidelines to follow are:

- Initially, one-piece outfits are recommended as they prevent the baby from pulling at the bag.
- Dresses and dungarees are best.
- A nappy must be sited below the stoma as any urine from the nappy (in the case of colostomies/ileostomies) or faecal matter (in the case or urostomates), may soil the bag.

Unwanted Baggage

- If you put pants over the nappy, the waistband must also be sited below the bag.

- Avoid stiff waistbands or belts.

- Avoid tight or clinging fabrics as these may catch obstruct free drainage and show the appliance.

- Avoid bare midriffs

- Ensure baby's nails are kept short so if they do mange to reach the bag they cannot tear it.

- You can make a small cotton band to cover the bag. – For the length, wrap material around baby so that it fits comfortably. Its depth should be that of the bag. Sew a hem at both ends and fix 3" Velcro tabs to hold in place. This can be easily then be adjusted easily as baby grows.

If you go out, always carry several spare bags and at least two sets of clothing with your nappy bag, Breast milk or formula may cause pockets of gas to form in the bag caused by air swallowed as the baby sucks. Check the bag regularly during feeding and release the gas to prevent the bag from bursting. Changing from milk to solids will be a time of trial and error. It is essential that you discuss feeding with the hospital dietician, as some foods will cause problems such as increased gas, liquid output etc. They will recommend a good diet and provide you with a list of foods that are not compatible with ostomies (such as nuts, vegetable skins etc.)

Fluid intake is extremely important for baby. Your consultant or GP will be able to recommend a daily fluid intake, over and above breast milk and formula. You should watch for signs of dehydration such as darkened urine of little urine output, listlessness, sunken eyes, lack of tears – call your stoma nurse of GP if you notice any of these signs as a young baby may become seriously dehydrated very quickly.

Day Care

Unfortunately, the majority of day-care centres may be unwilling or unable to take a very young ostomate. This is because the staff will not have been trained in emptying and changing a bag. (Per current Health & Safety regulations)Under health and safety guidelines, their own insurance policy may not cover them for caring for a child with an ostomy.

If you are looking for day-care for your child, your stoma nurse may be able to recommend a nursery in the area that has had experience. Once a child has reached the age when he or she can empty their own bag and possibly change with a little help, then a nursery may consider taking them.

Benefits

If you have to stay home and look after a child ostomate in receipt of DLA (all ostomates are entitled to **Disability Living Allowance**), then you qualify for a **Carer's Allowance**. Whilst this allowance is not equal to a full time wage, it does provide some extra finance to help with household expenses.

You may also be entitled to **Direct Payments** from your local Council to employ someone to help you with your child at home. Ask you local Social Services Team to conduct a Full Assessment., with this in mind. This applies as the child grows, keeping in mind that you will always have to be on hand to deal with any emergency.

Toddlers & the Older Child:

This is a time when along with potty training – you will start to teach you toddler to empty the bag. – Supervision is essential until your child reaches the age of 3-4. Always put a few sheets of toilet paper into the toilet basin, as this will prevent splash back. Lift the toilet seat and stand behind your child. Reach forward and show your child how to unfold the bag, extend it over the toilet and allow the contents to empty. Refold the bag, flush the toilet, and then wash hands. As a child grows more confident, you can stand aside as they manage to do this for themselves. They may get faecal matter on their clothes etc. but with patience, they will master this task. Allowing this to begin as early as feasibly possible will prepare them for doing this in nursery or school without help – and ensure their confidence in their ability.

Food is again an issue. There are certain foods that a child, as much as an adult, must not have as they may block the stoma; other foods, such as carbonated drinks, will cause gas. It is important to have a discussion with the hospital dietician, together with the child to ensure you both understand and avoid problems.

It is important for the child to understand you are not forbidding foods as a punishment, but rather that these foods may cause them serious harm. You will have to trust your child to attend parties and show restraint when these foods are presented. You can also explain that many children suffer from allergies and illnesses such as diabetes that also restrict what they can eat. You might want to set up a reward system to encourage healthy eating. This could also apply to siblings.

Fluid intake is very important. Child ostomates, particularly ileostomates, much drink an adequate amount of fluid for their age in relation to the type of ostomy. You will be able to get a specific chart from your consultant or dietician. Signs of dehydration include darkened urine, less urine output, listlessness, sunken eyes and no tears. A good hydration drink, such as pedialyte is excellent to supplement on a daily basis.

As a child grows, his or her curiosity will increase – clothing again may be an issue. Comfortable clothing is very important - If a child feels irritated by clothes rubbing over or against the stoma, they will become fretful.

- Use Velcro to adapt items of clothing that the child may perhaps be unable to wear.

- T-shirts with crotch snaps are ideal to prevent the toddler may discourage curious fingers

- Add an internal pocket at the level of the appliance to make wearing it more comfortable. This also decreases the likelihood of embarrassing accidents.

Unwanted Baggage

Going to School

The Government issues a number of publications and useful fact sheets which can assist with early and pre-schooling problems and other difficulties a parent may encounter when placing a disabled or chronically ill child in school'.

There are special schemes to support families with young children who are ill or for those with educational needs; including Early Support, Parent Partnership services and Home Visiting services see:
http://www.direct.gov.uk/en/Parents/Preschooldevelopmentandlearning/SpecialEducationalNeeds/DG_4000699

Staring school is always a great adventure. Starting school with an ostomy is no less of an adventure but will bring problems that other children will not have. It is essential that your child be able to change his or her bag without difficulty as accidents do happen! Talk about what might happen and how he or she will manage the situation.

Make a game of it and play "What if?" – "what if I need to go to the toilet because my bag is full?", "What if I have an accident?" etc. There are two very good leaflets produced by the Department of Health and the Council for the Disabled. These are "Every Child matters" for parents and "Including me" for children.

Another government website includes the above leaflets and much more information. As governments and policies change, then it is important to review this website regularly for any changes that may affect you.

www.everychildmatters.gov.uk

Under the **Disability Discrimination Act**, schools have legal responsibilities towards pupils with medical needs. Many pupils will actually fall into this category - nut allergies, hay fever, and diabetes and, while an ostomate pupil may be new to some schools, others will have had experience.

Medication that many ostomates have to take on a regular basis, together with problems in the absorption of nutrients may affect normal growth. This may mean that ostomates may be slightly smaller in height than their peers may. They may have to spend time away from school for treatment and hospitalisation. They may need to use the toilet urgently if they sense that the bag is full. They will need understanding with regard to gym classes, class outings etc. but children should be encouraged to take part in as many school activities as they feel able.

Your child should always carry spare bags and it is a good idea to keep a change of clothes at school in a locker or with the class teacher. You should alert the school that there will be days when he or she may not feel well enough to attend and you must ensure that missed lesson material is obtained promptly. Changing the bag takes time, so if a bag change is scheduled for the morning; try to make sure your child is not late for school, although you should alert the school that this may happen occasionally.

It is important to arrange an appointment with your child's designated class teacher, head teacher and whoever is in charge of PE or other classes that are taught by other teachers on a regular basis. It is important to do this

Unwanted Baggage

before school begins. You might like to ask your stoma nurse to accompany you, as teachers sometimes believe that a parent is being over-protective that is obviously not the case.

Some other questions that should be addressed are as follows:

- Initially, ask what the school's policies are with regard to children who have a medical condition. You can then review this together and ask any pertinent questions about this in general.

- If your child has to take medication during the school day, you should discuss how this could be handled. Break or lunch times are best so that he or she can meet with whoever is responsible for dispensing the medication outside of the classroom.

- Make sure that the school has all your contact numbers of where you can be reached at all times.

Discuss the exact nature of your child's need for privacy inasmuch as:

- They should be allowed to use a disabled toilet. If one is not available then the staff toilet/s should be made available to them.

- While not excluding your child from sport, swimming or PE, they should make separate changing arrangements, as they may be embarrassed about dressing and undressing wearing a bag. In addition, after any activity the bag may fill more quickly than usual requiring an immediate emptying or change in some circumstances. Schools will sometimes allow an ostomate to use a staff cloakroom or toilet. This is an essential arrangement.

- Your child should be able to leave a classroom as necessary, and if other teachers take over a class from time-to-time they should be made aware of this - perhaps choosing a seat near to the door might help a discreet exit.

- On outings, schools often appreciate parent volunteers so you may like to offer. You can suggest that your child be given an aisle seat on transport or at events and ask the teacher to track down the location of various toilets en route or at the destination.

After your child has been at school for a few weeks, you may suggest a review meeting to discuss how the school is managing. Your child may have brought up some issues, but it is important to hear the teacher's perspective on anything that may have happened.

It is important to encourage contact outside school with your child's classmates. Socialising with their peers will help prevent bullying. If at any time, you feel your child has been a target for ill-founded remarks or playground incidents then you must address this with the school as soon as possible, taking into consideration that most children undergo some kind of teasing during their school life and the extent to which these remarks may have upset your child.

Many children imagine themselves to be somehow different because they have a stoma. It is important to boost their confidence by stating the obvious – that a lot of people have something about them that makes them feel different – different colour hair, glasses diabetics are simple examples and explain that we do not like or dislike people for small differences. How boring would the world be if we were all identical? Talk about how they feel and discuss any problems, real or imaginary. At risk of repeating myself, communication is the most important tool in bringing up any child, with or without a stoma.

The Teen Years

These are trying times for any young person and perhaps more so for the teen ostomate. From a medical standpoint, some medications may delay puberty and even stunt growth – It is important that as a parent you should voice any concern you may have with both your GP and consultant, not forgetting of course to involve your teenager!

For most teens – body image is all. Dealing with acne is par for the course; dealing with an ostomy is different. Unfortunately, an ostomate has to make sensible clothing choices that may not be the height of fashion.

During a recent hospital stay, a justifiably grumpy teen was occupying a nearby bed with a crohn's flare-up. She was also an ostomate and, following the trend, had crammed herself and bag into a pair of jeans so tight, the bag had burst and she was mortified by the resultant accident. She also did serious damage due to the length of time she had been wearing these tight clothes. A dressing down by the consultant did little to ameliorate the situation. Fortunately, a good counsellor was on hand to talk her through what had happened and explore other equally fashionable items that could be worn as an alternate. She also thoughtfully arranged for her to have a makeover complete with new hairstyle and she was able to learn some great make-up tricks.

Your youngster will experience a gamut of feelings during their teen years – anger that they have to wear a bag; a sense of fear about accidents in public; more tests, and more treatment. They may feel embarrassed believing incorrectly that they "smell" or having to visit the toilet frequently. They may feel left out as they avoid the communal changing rooms and showers at sport functions. If a friend forgets to invite them to a group event, they may blame the stoma when it may be something else entirely.

Every teen confronts sexual issues. An ostomate teen will have additional questions from "When do I tell a friend I have an ostomy?", to the more physical question of "How to have sex with an ostomy?" (See section on intimacy). These questions may not mean that they actually intend to have sex but they will be curious. If they do not address these issues, you may want to bring them up yourself at an appropriate time.

A boyfriend or girlfriend may seem to tire of their ostomate friend. It will be so easy to "blame the ostomy"; instead

Unwanted Baggage

of realising that the teen years are a time of change, and of meeting new friends. Teen friends habitually come and go. Being "dumped" is a frequent teen experience and, in an ostomates' case, the bag will be seen as an easy scapegoat. Unfortunately, only time and new friends will help the situation. When your teen is obviously upset and miserable, a parent must be supportive and understanding but avoid constantly asking them how they are feeling. If they want to tell you, they will. The good thing about teens is that they do tend to bounce back.

Communication with any teenager is difficult but an ostomate may need external advice or counselling as it is so much easier to talk to a stranger than a family member. Do watch out for real warning signs – if a teen has led a good social life and suddenly retreats to a solitary existence behind a computer screen, refuses to go to family functions, becomes sullen, resentful or seem generally unhappy, then there is a real problem. Again, it is difficult to tell the difference between a normal sulky teen and an ostomate teen with more serious problems.

Exam time will bring stress. For some ostomates, their individual medical conditions may leave them susceptible to relapses or periods of exhaustion. You will need to help them find a balance between studying and staying fit. Coordinate with the school that will of course be able to re-schedule board examinations and may let them sit class exams at other times or at home. They can also arrange for board examinations to be sat in hospital.

Diet may become more of an issue – youngsters tend to hang out together and may involve large amounts of junk food or later alcohol or even drugs. Your teen should understand their individual dietary limitations. It is a good idea to schedule a meeting with the hospital dietician to discuss how they can fit in occasional junk food or drink without missing out on being "one of the crowd.". Discuss alcohol and drugs and the affects these can have on the ostomy and prescribed medications. Avoid saying they **MUST** avoid these, ask them what they think might happen if they happened to indulge. Ask them to read the contra-indicative information enclosed with their medications – that way they will realise what could happen. You could also ask your GP to address your concerns.

On the question of Rules, the teen ages are traditionally a time for rebellion. An ostomate child may have been slightly more cosseted that most children and may take advantage of this leniency to bend the house rules.

Treat your child as a normal teenager who has to follow rules about coming home on time, letting you know where they are, while affording them more privacy and understanding of their moods.

Fashion Advice for the teen

Head things off at the pass – they will be beginning to show their independence in choice of clothing but a little advice may go a long way to avoiding real problems:
- Baggy jeans are suitable for both sexes.
- A bodysuit for girls is comfortable and can provide extra support and discretion for the bag.

Unwanted Baggage

- Long t-shirts, worn with fashionable leggings are great for girls or with the baggy jeans for boys.

- For swimming or the beach: board shorts with a good lining are great for boys; Lycra underwear under a bathing suit for girls will hide a lot. Dependent upon operative scarring, a girl may be happier with a one-piece or tankini separates. A beautiful floaty chiffon top can complete a girl's beach outfit.

- Jean shorts can also be cut down from an old pair of comfortable denims. Jean fabric is excellent for swimming but it will stay wet longer. If a young man is sensitive about body scarring then they can swim in a t-shirt in the pool or at the sea. "Avoiding the sun", is a great excuse!

- Flowing dresses are ideal for special occasions.

- Comfortable underwear (see smugglingduds.com for underwear with a "bag" pocket) is essential. However, this does not have to mean baggy white cotton!! There are some lacy, pretty styles that are also feel great to wear. You can try the ostomy suppliers for great silk and lace garments or a size larger in briefs at conventional stores.

- A cami top is also a great lingerie addition.

- High waisted clothes are great.

Try to Avoid:

- Tight clothes – try all potential purchases on in front of a mirror and stand sideways to see if the bag shows. Keep the garment on for at least ten minutes; if it begins to feel uncomfortable then it is not for you.
- Lycra – except for underwear
- G-string undies
- Bare Midriff's or low slung jeans
- Tight jeans. Always, always take one size larger than you are
- Belts

Fortunately, there are some great ostomy websites especially for teens. They all have forums where they can meet other ostomates and exchange ideas.

Some of the forums are international and have facebook connections. Talking to another teen with an ostomy will make them realise that they are not alone.

Websites:

www.smiliespeople.org.uk
This is for families with a child or young person with IBD. Smilies Is a worldwide network focusing on the difficulties experienced by children who have IBD and their families. It gives them the opportunity to develop informal mutual support. You can join Smilies by becoming a member

of the **CROHN'S AND COLITIS UK.** They host an annual Christmas party, special Weekend Breaks and Family Fun Days that include dry slope skiing, ice skating, craft activities, circus visits, dancing, karaoke and swimming. Membership is free for young adults 16-18

www.crohnsandcolitisuk.org.uk
This National Association for Crohn's and Colitis is a good first contact point for parents of children who have either of these conditions that may lead to ostomies. They operate a "Parents to Parents" a telephone help service available to parents who have a child with IBD. This is an excellent first step resource.

www.home.vicnet.net.au/~youinc/welcome.htm
This is an Australian based International contact site for teens with ostomies and other intestinal/urological problems.

www.kidshealth.org
This website is for children aged 3-12, and it includes medical information - games and quizzes, recipes, hospital visits etc.

www.crohns4youngadults.co.uk
This is a great UK site for 10-14 yr olds with crohn's and those with ostomies. (Also called "Crohn's is Crap"). Lots of fun things to do and online youngsters to meet.

www.crohnszone.org
This is a fantastic all-ages chat and advice site for crohn's patients and ostomates. This site has an excellent forum section where you can exchange ideas on treatment and all sorts of ideas.

www.ostomy-winnipeg.ca/woa0905f.html
This is a moving story about a young teen with an ostomy. Any teen ostomate will relate to this.

www.pullthrunetwork.org
A support network (US based) for parents of children with ostomies and other bowel and urological disorders – lots of excellent advice and information.

www.teenibd.co.uk
A forum for teens with bowel diseases and ostomies – great website.

www.medikidz.co.uk!!!
This is without doubt my favourite website for children and young people with any illness. I even found it a good website to check on my own medication.

Millions of children worldwide are diagnosed every day with conditions that even their parents may find difficult to comprehend. Most children do not understand their medical conditions, or associated investigations, procedures and treatments, and are often scared by what is going on around them.

Traditionally, it was felt that children were too young to understand medical concepts, or even worse, were better off not knowing. Doctors often do not have the time or skills to explain medical issues, so that children and their families can understand them. There are over 50 million children in six main English-speaking countries that are currently afflicted with illness and are without proper educational resources. To date, no effective solution exists to this overwhelming global problem. There is therefore a definite, substantial and unsatisfied need in the marketplace for an offering like Medikidz. The best way to communicate with children is often through other children.

The 'Medikidz' are a gang of 5 larger-than-life superheroes from outer space, which are each specialists in different parts of the body. The characters are designed to be fun and appealing to children in order to be able to entertain, as well as educate them about serious medical issues. They are destined to become characters with whom children can relate, and befriend.

The Medikidz characters live on 'Mediland' - a living, moving planet shaped just like the human body. The children are taught about their own body by going on a personal tour through Mediland. Medikidz is designed specifically for children: therefore, it speaks their language, at their level, via comic books, games and an online virtual world.

Additional Resources for Parents and children
The Family Fund Trust
www.familyfund.org.uk
www.familyfundextra.co.uk

The family fund trust give grants for things that make life easier and more enjoyable for the disabled and chronically ill child and their family, such as washing machines, driving lessons, hospital visiting costs, computers and holidays. The Family Fund helps families with sick children to have choices and the opportunity to enjoy ordinary life.

Kids Days Out
www.kidsdaysout.co.uk
This is a directory of tourist attractions around the U.K, including whether or not they have accessible toilets. This is a great resource for everyone including families, school, outings, trips etc.

Action For Kids
www.actionforkids.org
Ability House
15A Tottenham Lane
Hornsey
London
N8 9DJ
Telephone: 020 8347 8111
Helpline: 0845 300 0237 (local call rates)
E-mail: info@actionforkids.org

This group helps disabled and chronically ill young people find more independence and opportunity through providing equipment and support.

They provide mobility aids, Work Related Learning (WRL) and offer family support services. They try never to say no and will help in any way they can to enable children and young people with health related problems and disabilities to lead full and independent lives.

3H Fund
www.3hfund.org.uk
B2 Speldhurst Business Park
Langton Road
Tunbridge Wells
Kent

TN3 0AQ
Telephone: 01892 860207
Grant Programme Telephone: 01892 860219

The 3H fund Organises subsidised group holidays for disabled and chronically ill children and adults to provide respite for their regular carers. It also provides some grants to families on low income with a disabled dependent.

Whizz-Kidz
www.whizz-kids.org.uk
1 Warwick Row
London
SW1E 5ER
Tel: 020 7233 6600
Email: info@whizz-kids.org.uk

Whizz-Kidz is all about giving disabled and chronically ill children and young people the independence to enjoy an active childhood at home, at school and at play.

By providing them with customised mobility equipment, training, advice and life skills, actually gives them something much more important - the independence to be themselves. We make an immediate and life changing difference to their lives and their families.

National Children's Bureau
www.ncb.org.uk
Established in 1963, the NCB is a charitable organisation that is dedicated to advancing the health and well-being of all children and young people across every aspect of their lives and providing them with a powerful and authoritative voice.

The NCB provides the latest information on policy, research and best practice across the sector as a whole; NCB offers essential support to those working with and on behalf of children, their families and carers.

Its young member's scheme, **Young NCB**, enables it to reach and support children and young people themselves, ensuring they are valued, their rights are respected and their voices can be heard.

Ability Net
www.abilitynet.org.uk
PO Box 94
Warwick
CV34 5WS
Tel: 01926 312847
Helpline: 0800 269 545
Email: enquiries@abilitynet.org.uk
Ability Net is a registered national charity with over 20 years experience helping people adapt and adjust their information and communications technology (ICT). Its special expertise is ensuring that whatever the age, health condition, disability or situation a person will find exactly the right way to adapt or adjust your ICT to make it easier to use.

There are a confusing number of adaptations that change frequently, and a huge range of prices. They will always point out the low cost and free solutions first and let you try various solutions, so you avoid making costly mistakes.

Computers for the Disabled, Chronically sick and Housebound.
www.cftd.co.uk/cftd.htm
This particular charity sources quality recycled PCs & new parts, which are then made available to the disabled, chronically ill, the housebound, and disabled centres etc.

Contact a Family
www.cafamily.org.uk/holidays
209-211 City Road
London
EC1V 1JN
Helpline: 0808 808 3555
Contact-a-Family provides support, advice and information for families with disabled or chronically sick children, no matter what their condition or disability. Contact a Family became a registered charity in 1979 and it has nearly 30 years of experience of working with families with sick children.

Breakaway
www.breakaway-visit.co.uk
email:break.away@tiscali.co.uk

Breakaway was started by Rachel Clarkson who was diagnosed with Crohn's disease in 2004, aged 28. Through www.ostomyland.com
she became friends with a young mother whose daughter had a colostomy at birth. They began to discuss the lack of support for parents and children with bowel or bladder dysfunctions and they decided to arrange a fun activity weekend for families to meet and share experiences and

have fun. That was in December 2008. Now they regularly organise activity weekends where children can take part in confidence building and action adventure activities. Stoma nurses are on hand to cope with any problems that may arise. A token charge is made, but funding is available for those with limited means.

College & University

For young adults living away from home is a new and exciting adventure. Just because you have a stoma does not make it any less of an experience. Most colleges and universities prefer their students to live on campus for their first year. At older established institutions, halls of residence were an afterthought (apart from some Oxford and Cambridge), as such, they are dotted hither and thither all over the nearest town. Some offer shared accommodation; the more modern colleges have small campus villages. Whatever your scenario, it is a good idea to visit the location well beforehand; perhaps taking advantage of an "Open Day", to explore the terrain and choose the best option for your situation.

Ensure that you put in an application as soon as possible to ensure you get your first choice. You can talk to the Student Support team at the college to ask that they give priority to your choice on medical grounds. During your visit, have a good look for the location of campus toilets and look at the menus on the campus catering. This will help you choose between catered of self-catering halls of residence.

There is a superb guide to facilities and life on campus for disabled and chronically ill students. **"The Disabled Students' Guide to Universities" by Emma Caprez.** The 2005 edition seems to be the latest but check with websites such as Amazon.co.uk who are offering this at £0.62 plus postage £2.75 for used copies. Do not be put off by the "disabled" tag – it is a helpful look at facilities and provides excellent advice for stoma patients.

Disabled Students' Allowances (DSAs)

DSAs provide extra financial help to students with a disability, ongoing health condition, mental health condition or learning difficulty. The grants differ from England to Wales and Scotland who have their own individual programs.

DSA grants to help meet extra course costs that students can face because of their individual conditions. They are paid in addition to the student finance package – the amount depends on your individual circumstances – not on household income.

The grants can help fund specialist equipment, non-medical helpers, extra travel costs, dietary needs and extra clothing costs that you may incur as you may have to return home for hospital appointments or for rest periods. You have to be eligible for student finance to qualify for DSA's . It is important to check with the websites listed below as each area offers different amounts for different needs. These may change dependent upon year of entry. Stoma patients are eligible for the general category including dietary/clothing and travel expenses.

See:
www.direct.gov.uk/en/DisabledPeople/ EducationAndTraining/HigherEducation/DG_10034898
- England

www.studentfinanceni.co.uk/portal/page?_ pageid=54,1268397&_dad=portal&_schema=PORTAL
– Northern Ireland

www.saas.gov.uk/_forms/slc_terms_conditions_1011. pdf
- Scotland

www.studentfinancewales.co.uk/portal/ page?_pageid=56,1275855&_dad=portal&_ schema=PORTAL#section3 - Wales

Medical Assistance

You may wish to retain your local GP or alternatively register with the University Health Service. The UHS may suggest that you register instead with a local doctor. It is important to discuss your options with them. Your gastroenterologist or urologist may suggest a local hospital or consultant so that your records, or a copy thereof, can be transferred ahead of time. You may of course decide to remain with your local medical facilities and travel for regular appointments.

Emergencies may occur but if you have a copy of your medical records this will save time in treating you if the need arises. Your should alert your medical supply company that you need to register two addresses for

Unwanted Baggage

your deliveries or continue to have them delivered to your home and collect them as necessary. This may well save embarrassment but also of these getting lost in the massive student postal system. Keep a record of your prescriptions and medical supplies handy so you can telephone for repeats.

Coursework & Exams

On arrival at college, you will be assigned a personal tutor or counsellor. It would be sensible to advise them of your medical conditions and discuss anything you think may interfere with your studies. You should explain that you may sometimes need to leave a lecture to visit the toilet (make sure you sit near an exit so that you can leave discreetly). There is a certain amount of stress for anyone starting college – this may manifest itself as a flare-up or a general feeling of being unwell.

If you need to miss a class to rest then you must do so. You can always explain to the lecturer later and obtain the necessary coursework. (You are entitled to coursework extensions in the event of ill health). Your personal tutor may be able to arrange automatic extensions as periods of hospitalisation or medical rest needs occur. Do discuss the possibility of events occurring with your tutor, rather than leave them to after the fact. You are not making excuses for yourself. You have genuine reasons to miss studies and providing you do not exploit this, your teaching staff will understand fully.

University examinations are serious. They are also a time of stress. Stress can cause bags to fill more quickly than usual and may result in you having to leave the hall to avoid an accident.

The administration of these examinations is taken very seriously by the universities. Arrive early at the examination hall and make sure that the adjudicator knows you may have to visit the toilet urgently. You should pre-arrange a signal to alert them if it becomes necessary. Sit near the exit so that you can leave quietly. In some instances, you may have to provide a medical certificate to an independent adjudicator and you may even be assigned someone to accompany you to and from the toilet. This is standard practice; you are not being singled out.

If you are admitted to hospital during examination, alert the university, who will make special arrangements for you to take it either in hospital or at a later date,

Party Time!

University life is not all about work. It is a time of meeting new people, making new friends and enjoying your new found independence. At home, your old friends may have known about your illness and understood the self-imposed restrictions of diet and your need to maintain a low level of alcohol consumption. Your parents will have been there to guide you and like it or not, monitored your behaviour in regard to both. Now you are on your own and it is up to you alone to be cautious of what you eat or drink. No one is trying to dampen the party spirit, but too much indulgence will seriously affect your health. It is easy to say, but confronted with *Fresher's Week* and

Unwanted Baggage

organised *Pub Crawls,* the reality becomes so much more difficult.

Rather than having to explain why you are not knocking them back with the best of them, you can do a few sensible things. Buy your own drinks – or make sure you fill the order for you and your friends. That way you can order sparking water with a twist and call it gin and tonic; a simple coke can be described as a "mixer". You can always pretend you are recovering from the night before or even a stomach flu. That way you will not call attention to yourself.

Keep on the alert for anything that is bought for you. People always try to be clever. A drink may contain several different types of spirit, disguised by the taste of coke – vodka and coke is hardly discernible from plain coke to the taste or smell. Sip the drink slowly, if you are at all suspicious, in the crowd discreetly put the remains down somewhere else.

Other people have to restrict what they drink too – people with diabetes are prime examples and many others are teetotal on religious grounds, you are not alone. Eventually your friends will come to know that you have a medical condition that does not react well to large amounts of alcohol. You will then be welcomed as the designated driver!

The party mood also brings with it a certain amount of sexual energy. Be aware that the contraceptive pill does not work if you have a colostomy or ileostomy. Do carry condoms for the "heat of the Moment". Smuggling Duds (smugglingduds.com) are an excellent source of underwear with a built-in pocket to carry a spare bag and condoms discreetly under jeans without the need for a bulky emergency pack. Most universities have a contraceptive advice service that will offer advice and help as necessary.

Where there is a university there is a drugs scene. Be aware that if you are taking medication of any kind, any other drugs may react badly with it. Cocaine, Heroin, Ecstasy. Methamphetamines or the new designer drugs have potentially lethal reactions when taken with prescribed medication. If you take any of these substances or think that someone may have slipped you something, then you must seek medical help immediately.

Advice and Counselling

Do not be afraid to ask for advice or help at any time. Each university and College has a dedicated team to help students with any problems no matter how small. However, it is up to you to seek them out and freely discuss your concerns. No problem is insurmountable and these dedicated people are there to ensure that your life at university is an enjoyable culmination of all your hard efforts at school. Whatever your situation, someone somewhere will have been in the same position before. For every problem, there is a solution.

Your parents will be overly concerned for you. It is important to communicate with them – arrange to call once a week – or just send regular emails. If you are unhappy, go home for the weekend, spend a few days with old friends and enjoy spending time with your family

Unwanted Baggage

– they will be delighted to see you and you will return refreshed.

Other useful Student websites

Skill: The National Bureau for Students
With Disabilities
www.skill.org.uk
Email: info@skill.org.uk

Chapter House
18-20 Crucifix Lane
London
SE1 3JW
Helpline: 0800 328 5050
SKIL is a national charity promoting opportunities for young people and adults with any kind of impairment or illness in post-16 education, training and employment.

Skill also advises of your rights to study while receiving disability or incapacity benefits.

This is an excellent resource to begin research into further education and employment opportunities. It offers a number of grants from potential employers who regularly recruit disabled and chronically ill students.

Examination Hiccups
www.cs3.brookes.ac.uk/student/services/health/exam.html

This is a wonderful guide to managing examination stress for all students – ostomates or not!.

Dance Safe
www.dancesafe.org

Great website to plan what to take to a rave and other details on dance locations and information etc.

The Site
www.thesite.org

This is a really good site for all 18-25 yr olds on every possible topic – drugs, relationships, studies, stress, the law, money issues - excellent advice and further resources/links.

Chapter Nineteen
Ostomical Workplace
... Returning to, or starting work with an ostomy

Before the Ostomy

Prior to your operation, you will have experienced periods of time when you have been unable to work due to the illness that has caused your consultant to plan an ostomy. During this period, you may have taken days off work due to your health for which you should have received Statutory Sick pay from your employer. This period may overlap with the recovery period from surgery. If you have not applied for SSP then you are entitled to do so for the recovery period.

Statutory Sick Pay (SSP)

SSP is paid if you have a contract of employment (even if you have only just started.
- You are sick for at least four days in a row (including weekends and bank holidays).
- You are earning more than £97.00 per week.

- If you have more than one employer, you may claim SSP from each employer.

- You will receive SSP from your employer on your normal payday.

- Employers may operate their own sick day scheme in addition to or in place of SSP. The details of this will be included in your contract of employment.

- You are entitled to 28 weeks of SSP. If this comes to an end and you continue to be off work, then your employer must give you form SSP1 for you to claim Employment and Support Allowance that will be paid by the DWP

If you continue to be unemployed after 28 weeks, then you will have to apply for Employment & support Allowance bearing in mind the following:

After the Ostomy...

Returning to your old employer

It is always better to err on the side of caution. If you are worried about when you should return to work, initially you should consult with your doctor and stoma nurse as they can help you make an informed decision.

If your work consisted or any heavy lifting or arduous manual work, you must discuss your current abilities with your GP to allow him to gauge whether or not you will be able to continue in this field, or what appliances are available to protect the stoma and any danger of hernia damage that such strenuous work may cause.

Other guidelines before organising a date for your return:

- You must be able and comfortable with changing your bag and be used to dealing with any small emergencies that can occur – leakage, ballooning etc.

- You feel that your energy is returning and you will be able to cope with the normal stresses and strains of work life.

- You are ready to travel/drive

- You are entirely comfortable in the company of others. While you will be conscious of wearing a bag, it is important not to keep checking it. If you are concerned, pop to the toilet regularly to reassure yourself that all is well. After a few weeks, these concerns will pass.

It is a good idea to have a dry run, plan a day before your scheduled return, arrive at work and test the waters. If things do not go as you hoped, give it another few weeks and try again. Building up your confidence slowly without forcing yourself to rush into a return to normal work, routines will help. Most employers will be very empathetic and work with you.

Benefits

If you are claiming **SSP** and wish to return to work gradually, you will have to get a letter from your GP to the effect that the work is initially of therapeutic value. You will then continue to receive this benefit until you are working a full work week. This process is recognised by the DWP. You must not work in excess of 15.99 hours in any one week to continue claiming it.

New Welfare Reform Bill announced:

The Queen's speech announces a new <u>Welfare Reform Bill</u> that will scrap all existing back to work programmes and establish a single welfare-to-work regime. All incapacity benefit claimants will also be reassessed. *The current situation as of June 2010 is as follows:*

Employment & Support Allowance

Employment and support allowance has replaced Incapacity Benefit. The application form is complex (although the new government has promised to simply these forms), so do not hesitate to ask for help with this. It is designed to assess your ability to work at the time of application and, based on the information provided, how it will affect your future ability to work. ESA will then provide excellent support as and when you are able to return to work. You are also allowed to do "permitted work" while still claiming ESA . For exact details see:
<u>www.direct.gov.uk/en/DisabledPeople/ FinancialSupport/esa/DG_171894</u>

Disability Living Allowance (DLA)

Even if you are employed, as an ostomate, you are entitled to Disability Living Allowance in addition to your earnings.

Extras

When you return to work, remember to carry with you an emergency change kit with at least three spare bags. You may also wish to keep a change of underwear/clothes in case of a sudden leakage. These can be stored in a desk or locker. Remember to allow yourself a good ten minutes to empty your bag at least three times during the day. If you are taking medication, then remember to keep this on your person, in a handbag or in a locked drawer. You are liable for any medication in your possession or prescribed to you. As hydration is paramount for all ostomists, ensure you have access to a drink at all times. Tea is as hydrating as water but coffee is not. A bottle of water is always a good standby.

New Employment Opportunities

It may be that you find yourself unable to cope with your former job, or your employer may not understand your needs to spend a little longer than average in the restroom. They may be overly concerned that your stoma will affect your work, and, whilst this may be untrue, their attitude may make you feel unwelcome or out of place.

You may have been employed in a job that requires physical or manual activity that you are no longer permitted to do. This may be personal choice, medical advice or under your employer's health and safety regulations.

Whatever the reason, if you are worried about returning to the same employment for any reason, you should arrange an appointment to speak with the **Disability Employment Officer** at the local Job Centre. They will be happy to seek alternative employment for you in a workplace better suited to your needs. There are many incentives for employers (and employees) to take on a person with difficulties or disabilities. The DEO will also offer any retraining that you might need.

A "Disability Officer" may sound ominous, but they work on a day-to-day basis with employers who operate an equal opportunities charter. These companies must employ 10% "disabled" as part of their workforce. You are an attractive prospect to an employer who may be surprised to find that you in fact take less sick time than non-disabled members of staff do.

Employers may agree to take you on a trial basis for six weeks to see if the new arrangement suits both of you. In this case, the Government will pay 45% per week of your wage to your employer (who pays the other 55%). If you both concur that all is well at the end of this period and you are happy in your new environment, then your employer will offer a full time contract.

Legal Requirements

There are legal requirements that employers must observe in respect of disabled employees.

Since October 2004, all employers must apply all sections of the Disability Discrimination Act (DDA). This applies to all firms, regardless of the number of employees they have. The goal of the DDA legislation is stop discrimination against employed disabled people applying for work or people training for work. The DDA also covers those in temporary or contractual employment and those on work placements. The only exceptions to employers under the DDA are the armed forces.

The results of any severe illness and consequent operations leave patients with differing abilities. You may not like the use of the word "disabled" as a classification. The DDA considers you to be disabled if you have **'a physical or mental impairment which has a substantial and long-term adverse effect on your ability to carry out normal day-to-day activities'**. This term is applied to people who are deaf, have movement problems, skin diseases, asthma, epilepsy, people who have had successful heart surgery and yes, those with stomas are included in the Government catalogue of "disabilities".

While you may be confident that you are able to carry out any task an employer may ask of you, the causes of stomas, e.g. Crohn's, Colitis, Cancers etc. may bring about other problems (regular GP or hospital appointments, flare-ups, extreme bouts of diarrhoea, abdominal pains, occasional re-hospitalisation and days when you have an lack of energy). These ancillary problems may interfere with your work schedule. Having a stoma is a life-changing operation. It puts you in the disabled classification for employment purposes that enables an employer to understand that when they employ you, there may be days when you are not able to work. Acceptance of this classification, allows you to be a responsible employee affording you the opportunity to work as well as you can, when you can.

On those occasions when you are unwell, Under the DDA rules, your employer should fully understands and allows for these instances. Under these circumstances, your colleagues too, should make uncritical allowances for your absences and help you catch up on your return.

In seeking and maintaining employment, you have a great deal of protection under the DDA. The Act maintains that Employers must not:

- Directly discriminate against a disabled person.
- Treat an employee less favourably for a reason related to their disability, without good reason.

Employers must also make reasonable adjustments in all of aspects of employment, working conditions or the workplace to enable or assist you to do a job.

What is considered 'reasonable' always depends on individual circumstances. Adjustments could include physical changes to the workplace – i.e. grab rails, stair

Unwanted Baggage

lifts, or more importantly for an ostomate is an accessible toilet.

Larger companies may have a number of disabled employees and therefore may do more to change the workplace than smaller companies would. However, all employers must show that are prepared to make necessary changes. In many cases, local and national government funding is available. The Jobcentre will provide details of all possible adaptations and sources of funding.

An employer may not reject a job application on the grounds of disability. If you declare your disability and feel that you have been discriminated against during the application process, you can take your concern to an employment tribunal.

You must also take into account that it is illegal to give false information on any work application. Most job application forms and accompanying medical questionnaires require you to give details about your health. If you do not give the correct information, you could be liable for dismissal.

When discussing your disability with your potential employer, you should use positive strategies to emphasise your skills. Rather than telling a prospective employer 'I have a stoma and associated illness which may cause problems', you could say 'Because of my illness, I have developed a great deal of patience that has enhanced my ability to concentrate. This allows me to perform complex, detailed tasks'. Emphasise that you feel well enough to work full (or part time as the case may be).

By highlighting any potential difficulties that you may have and showing the ways you can overcome them will show maturity and determination. As an ostomate you should tell an employer that you might need extra time to use the toilet but that your will pay close attention to your timekeeping and make up any time missed by arriving early or departing later than your standard hours.

During an interview, Employers may:

- Not ask candidates irrelevant health questions.

- Only ask questions about disability before making a job offer if they relate to the recruitment process

- Provide a health questionnaires relating to a particular job.

- Only carry out a health assessment after a job offer is made.

If A Disability Officer has recommended you, the Employer should have a full understanding of the situation.

Once employed, your employer must provide (may already have) an accessible toilet that contains a toilet, shelf and sink with hot and cold water. It is important that your employer is fully aware of your toilet needs and makes provision for a chemical waste bin/disposal service so that your pouches can be hygienically disposed of without risk to other employees. Your employer must keep your condition confidential. It is up to you whether you to choose to inform your colleagues.

Unwanted Baggage

Retraining

If you have to seek a change of career, you might also want to consider retraining. One of the finest <u>funded</u> residential training institutions that focus on the needs of the disabled is the Queen Elizabeth's Foundation. It offers a variety of courses from bookkeeping to vehicle spray painting. All courses include travel and accommodation. For more information contact:

The Queen Elizabeth's Foundation
<u>www.qef.org.uk</u>
Queen Elizabeth's Foundation
Woodlands Road, Leatherhead Court
Leatherhead
Surrey
KT22 0BN
Tel: 01372 841100
Email: <u>info@qef.org.uk</u>

The Queen Elizabeth's Foundation encourages and enables adults with disabilities to increase independence and improve life skills. The Foundation's aim is to ensure that all adults in the United Kingdom with disabilities, chronic illness, or those with mental or physical problems can access the training and support required to achieve their goals. The Queen Elizabeth's foundation

- Is funded by Jobcentre Plus, part of the Department of Work and Pensions. The Residential Training Unit manages the contract.

- Trainees who are on state benefits: .SSP, Income Support or Job Seeker's Allowance, will continue to receive the same rate of benefit whilst on training (with the exception of any "Care" component, which will be lost during residency at QEF).

- Trainees being referred from any other source, including direct referrals will be accepted subject to assessment and agreement on funding.

- Funding covers the costs of your actual training, equipment and/or protective clothing needed for your training, accommodation and full board.

For applicants referred through Jobcentre Plus:

- You must be over 18 years of age.

- You must have an on-going health problem or disability.

- You must be unemployed before your training starts.

- Your goal should be employment, either open or supported, or self-employment, on completion of training.

- You must have a good prospect of employment in the chosen training occupation in your home area.

The QEF is a little known resource and your local Job Centre's Disability Officer may not have heard of it. This is not unusual, so print out the course(s) you are

Unwanted Baggage

most interested in and take the details with you to the Jobcentre. They then will ask you to complete a CV and a brief summary of why you want to pursue the course and resultant job opportunities that you think would be available on completion. They will then forward everything to the DWP for approval (a rubber stamp exercise, if your Disability Officer thinks it is a good idea). Funding will then be made available to QEF who will send you their own application form for final approval and start date. Courses are only residential but travel home is funded from Thursday – Monday, every two weeks for the duration of the course. The QEF has several open days and it would be a good idea to visit the institute before deciding on these courses.

Other Resources

If you are seeking to train for other careers there are a number of free residential courses open to disabled students of any age. For more information look at:

www.direct.gov.uk/en/DisabledPeople

And:

www.direct.gov.uk/en/DisabledPeople/ Employmentsupport/WorkSchemesAndProgrammes/ DG_4011789

Employment Opportunities for People with Disabilities www.opportunities.org.uk

If you want expert advice of finding a job, the website is a good place to start. It is a national charity dedicated to creating routes into employment for people with all disabilities and medical conditions. In the last 10 years, alone, it has helped over 10,000 people towards work.

The Disability Alliance
www.disabilityalliance.org

This excellent resource can advise on benefit applications, job opportunities or any difficulty you might encounter in the workplace, training institution, or with DWP communication etc.

The Diversity Group
www.thediversitygroup.co.uk

The Diversity Group was established in 2006. Its aims are to eliminate barriers within employment, education and training for minority groups within the UK. It organises its own recruitment fairs throughout the UK. It maintains stands at disability and ethnic events in order to provide a service to prospective employees/employers.

The Diversity Group's primary objective is to promote equal opportunities to people from every kind of minority background or lifestyle, including race, gender, disability, age, faith and sexual orientation.

It maintains an active jobsite, offering employment nationwide. You can register free with your CV or just apply for one of the online job offers.

The Disabled Living Foundation
www.dlf.org.uk

This website offers general advice on benefit problems and links for those with difficulties in returning to work. It also has an impartial equipment advisory service.

Chapter Twenty
Leaving work
... Retiring, ill health, or to become a full or part-time carer

---

Unfortunately, it is very common that the illnesses that caused the ostomy have led to other symptoms that, combined with ostomy surgery may result in being left with limited mobility or other conditions ill suited to a workplace.

Cancers and Crohn's disease particularly linked with ME or fibromyalgia cause lethargy, exhaustion and depression. Medication, such as Methotrexate injections, can also have serious side effects preventing work. Medications may also be classified as "Do not Drive or Operate Machinery while under this prescription medicine. Thus, you may not be able to reach your workplace, let alone operate the machinery necessary to do the job.

Ostomy surgery itself can also leave to serious cases of depression. You can be left feeling frustrated and angry because you are not able to do those things that you want to do, let alone, work. Your Carer may be forced to leave work to care for you adding to your feelings of dependency and general uselessness. I speak from personal experience of all those things, when I say I know how you feel! Not to be able to make your body do

Unwanted Baggage

what you want is more than just frustrating. It is also remarkable to realise that a chronic illness can also wreak havoc on concentration and motivation.

Following surgery, take comfort that the operation is behind you; that the post-operative care is usually that of the highest possible calibre. Plenty of visitors, family and friends indulge your every whim. You have plenty of company, continued visits from the Stoma and District Nurses. However, after that passes and visitors return to their normal lives, you will find that the days get longer despite the best concerns and attention from those close to you. Your reliance on a carer may only underscore your lack of purpose. It is at these times that you will need to make plans.

You now have two choices. One, you can, as I stated in the chapter on emotions, allow yourself the privileges of becoming a true invalid, waited on hand and foot sinking into the depths of boredom and apathy. If you are reading this, then that is not the life for you. Option two: As self-pity should be limited, Your friends and family will soon tire of hearing the same old story.

Yes, there will be days when you are feel really unwell and cannot do much at all. Indulge yourselves on those days and rest as much as possible for that is what your body is telling you to do. On those days when you feel even slightly energised find an activity to do – reading, writing, painting, knitting, learning a new hobby, brush up your laptop skills etc.

The simplest form of mobility is ANY mobility. Keep the blood flowing. Ask your occupational therapist about simple exercises, even those that can be done in bed.

On those days that you are well enough to leave the house, do so. Even a hospital appointment is a reason to venture out into the world.

One of the most useful experiences is it to join a support group. The three main ostomy associations all have local groups with regular meetings where you can exchange ideas, make new friends and most importantly compare notes.

Talking to someone who has gone through the same procedure, has similar problems and especially those who are progressing well, is a definite soul-booster. The hints and tips you will acquire through conversation and invited speakers bring positive thinking about what you can achieve.

If new treatment regime is prescribed, you can ask others who may be already receiving it to give you their thoughts. The groups may host social events from coffee mornings to outings. At this point, I would like to thank all the members of Crohn's and Colitis UK, Aberystwyth Branch for their friendship, care and concern and support to both my husband and myself. Our time with them has been really enjoyable and informative and I hope will continue for many years.

If the breadwinner chooses to become the ostomate's carer then decisions have to be made. A part-time Carer may be able to work flexible hours or work from home.

A full time carer may also work from home (15.99hr permitted work per week to remain in receipt of benefits). Whatever the choice, discuss it with Social Services.

Crohn's and Colitis UK
(formerly: National Association for Colitis and Crohn's Disease)
www.Crohn's and Colitis UK.org.uk
4 Beaumont House
Sutton Road
St Albans
Hertfordshire
AL1 5HH
Telephone: 0845 1302233

Crohn's and Colitis UK is one of the largest groups with over 70 groups nationwide (and more beginning on a regular basis). They also run a hotline, parents' advice line and have a fantastic website with all the latest medical and other support information.
There is always someone to talk to on any subject.

They are the most approachable society I have ever encountered and use less of their fundraising income on personnel than any other charity I know. Their income goes towards essential research, welfare and events. Do not hesitate to join them if your have IBD.

The Colostomy Association
www.colostomyassociation.org.uk
2 London Court
East Street
Reading
Berkshire
RG1 4QL
Telephone: 0118 939 1537
Helpline: 0800 328 4257

The primary role of the Colostomy Association is to represent the interests of people with a colostomy.

It offers practical information for colostomates and people about to undergo surgery. Twenty-four hour helpline and 70 volunteers based nationwide to make home and hospital visits to members on request.

The Ileostomy and Internal Pouch Support Group
http://www.iasupport.org
Peverill House
1-5 Mill Road
Ballyclare
BT39 9DR
Telephone: 0800 0184724

IA, the Ileostomy and Internal Pouch Support Group (formerly known as the Ileostomy Association of Great Britain and Ireland), is a mutual support group that has the primary aim of helping people who have had their colon removed.

They have 55 regional groups throughout the UK and Eire who provide contact and meeting points for all ileostomists.

Urostomy Association
www.urostomyassociation.org.uk
Buckland
Beaumont Park
Danbury
Essex
CM3 4DE
Telephone: 01245 224294

UA assists those who are about to undergo or who have undergone surgery which results in a urinary diversion, such as a urostomy, continent urinary pouch or neo bladder.

It has 17 support branches throughout the UK who organise regular support meetings.

NASPCS National Advisory Service for Parents of Children with Stomas
secretary: Mr John Malcolm
51 Anderson Drive,
Valley View Park,
Darvel,
KA17 0DE
Scotland
Telephone: :01560 322024 51
No known website. Please correspond through letter of telephone.

Elizabeth Prosser & Philip Prosser

Children with Crohn's and Colitis
www.cicra.org

Martina Gaffney,
Charity Co-ordinator at CICRA,
Parkgate House, 356
West Barnes Lane,
Motspur Park,
Surrey, KT3 6QJ
Telephone 020 8949 6209

CICRA is dedicated to creating a wider understanding of Crohn's Disease and Ulcerative Colitis, collectively known as inflammatory bowel disease (IBD), particularly as it affects children and young adults.

Chapter Twenty One
Pregnancy and Childbirth
... *Yes, you Can!*

The study, **'Pregnancy, *delivery, and postpartum experiences of women with ostomies'*** , By Rupert B. Tuurbull, Jr. School of ET Nursing, Cleveland Clinic Foundation, Ohio. showed that Stoma (only) related problems that did not affect the foetus, during the second or third trimester were reported by 68.5% of patients. However, these problems were corrected without medical intervention. Solutions related to bag placement and adhesion and some blockages. The conclusions of the report stated: *"The presence of an ostomy should not be a deterrent to successful pregnancy and delivery. Having a Colostomy will not affect your ability to become pregnant. "*

Teamwork between your GP, gastroenterologist and gynaecologist will be essential during an ostomate's pregnancy. However, as an ostomist, you should not have trouble during pregnancy arising from your Stoma.

An immediate plus is no haemorrhoids! An Ileostomist runs a slightly greater risk of her Stoma experiencing partial blockages due to pressure exerted on the intestine. When the abdomen becomes distended during the later months, you may experience colicky pain. If this happens and lasts for more than a few hours then immediately ask your specialists for their advice. If this persists then a liquid diet may be recommended. In severe cases, hospitalisation may be necessary to ensure that both you and your baby receive adequate nutrition.

Maintaining an adequate fluid level is very important, especially if you suffer from morning sickness. You must keep drinking no matter what and consult your GP if you are at all worried about dehydration. If you suffer from morning sickness, try to eat little and often avoiding rich or greasy foods.

Urostomists are prone to infection during pregnancy, so again, drinking lots of water is important. If you think you have a urinary infection, consult your GP immediately. Luckily, urostomists do not experience additional urine in the bag than normal during pregnancy (frequent urination is common to most normal pregnancies due to pressure on the bladder).

As your abdomen enlarges, you may experience leakage, it is important to watch the stoma careful and apply extra flanges as necessary to keep the bag in place.

Antenatal Classes

If you take part in antenatal classes, it is important to let the person running the class know that you have a stoma. Do take changes of bags and clothes in case of bag disasters. Always change your bag after the class as the exercises may have weakened the bag's seals.

During pregnancy, it is likely that your Stoma will change shape. If this happens you need to be sure your appliance still fits properly. Ask your Stoma Nurse to check this for you every month and be prepared to change to a different brand/size of appliance if necessary.

Ultrasound Examinations

During an ultrasound, the large amounts of fluid that they use may seep under the bag seals. After the examination has finished, you should change the bag. Pregnant mothers are normally asked to drink a lot of fluid and refrain from going to the toilet before an ultrasound. This is because a full bladder gives a clear view of the baby. Urostomists may experience problems in getting a good ultrasound, but be reassured by the constant heartbeat, that the baby is fine.

As the pregnancy progresses, scans may be complicated by the position of a baby in relation to the stoma. If the baby's head is beneath the stoma, It will be difficult to get any accurate measurements. Babies move a lot in the womb so arrange an alternate appointment in the hope that he or she will have positioned themselves differently. If not, then ask for a vaginal scan that is a good alternative. Again, your gynaecologist will advise you if they think there are any problems.

Delivery

When you prepare your hospital bag for yourself and the baby, make sure you pack sufficient stoma supplies for your stay. With luck, you will deliver the baby in the same hospital at which your Stoma Nurse is based. That way you can be visited regularly by the Nurse to have the stoma checked, just as you did when you had the ostomy.

Whichever way the baby is delivered, you'll need to change the appliance as soon as possible afterwards as the stoma will swell due to the pressure and strain exerted during delivery. The attendant midwife or nurses may do this for you during labour (and immediately afterwards if you are unable to do this yourself). Make sure you take your bag supplies into the delivery room.

If during your original ostomy surgery, the rectum was removed, leaving scar tissue between the vagina and the original site of the anus, it may be necessary to do an episiotomy enlarging the vaginal entrance, in order to make the birth easier and prevent tearing. Episiotomies are as common in women who have rectums. If the removal of the rectum has caused nerve damage to the surrounding area, you may have to resort to a delivery by Caesarean section. If your gynaecologist thinks you will need a Caesarean, then it will be discussed with you in advance.

Unwanted Baggage

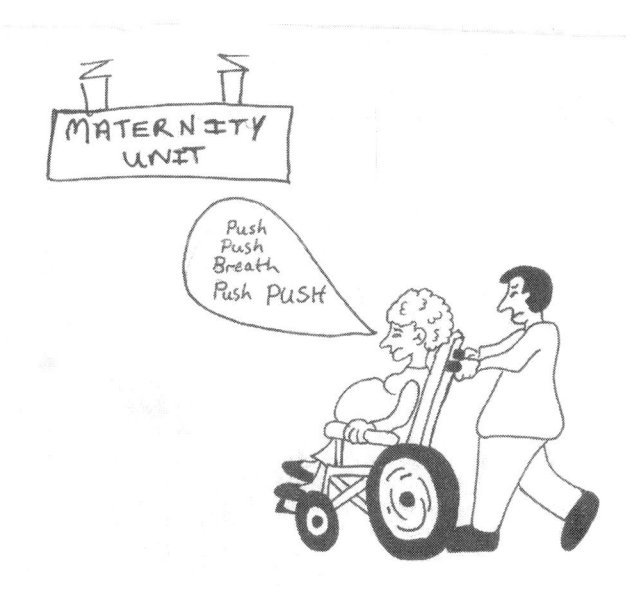

Post Partum

After the birth, you will be able to breastfeed as normal if you wish. No future pregnancies will be affected. Your stoma however, will give you a few problems as you shrink back to your original size. Ensure that you keep in regular contact with your stoma nurse and you may have to alter the bags or add seals as the process of returning to normal proceeds. After about three months, your stoma should return to its normal size.

Useful website:

Disabled pregnancy and parenthood
www.dppi.org.uk
Telephone: 08000184730
This site contains Information on pregnancy and parenthood for people who are disabled or with chronic illnesses.

Chapter Twenty two
Caring
... Life as a Carer

By Philip Prosser

I have no medical background, yet suddenly I found myself with the responsibility, the well-being, and basically, the life of another person in my hands. We, as carers, accept these grave responsibilities because of our feelings, our love, or perhaps out of duty, friendship, or guilt. Whatever the reason, there is only one certainty - your life will change.

This simply means that life will not be for the worst or for the better but rather a change in its direction. You will find qualities in yourself you never realised you had. You will face and deal with problems you never thought you were able to. There will be dark times that you will have to share with the person for whom you are caring. Even these can form a new type of bond and understanding between you both.

There are so many different situations and circumstances that play a part in the way in which you "care" These are:

- **Type and severity of the illness**: This will affect the way in which you care and the time that you devote to your patient.

- **Age of the patient:** The way in which you care and the amount of additional help you can receive will depend on whether you are caring for a child or an older patient.

- **Mobility of the patient:** Dependent upon the patient's ability to move around, will determine your own status. You may not be able to leave the house without arranging for special transport or someone to remain in the house while you are out.

- **Health and age of the carer:** If you are no longer a spring chicken, your own abilities may be limited.

- **Your financial circumstances**: If the main or sole breadwinner becomes ill or gives up their job to become the carer, you may find that your financial position has completed altered.

- **Amount of time you can devote:** You may find that while you have to care for a sick child, healthy siblings also need your attention. A couple may find themselves caring for each other in different ways.

- **Travel & Medical and Social Care**: The distance you have to travel for medical care; your relationship with the doctors and staff you encounter. The help you receive from

Unwanted Baggage

>social services in adaptations and other support services.

It is a fact that a patient with a supportive and understanding carer will enjoy a better quality of life. There is clear evidence that patients also respond and improve with such support. While there are no magic formulae or golden rules to follow you, as a carer, must remember that you are just as important as the person is in your care. Like an expectant mother "eating for two", as a carer you are caring for two, the patient and yourself.

If you financial circumstances have become strained because of you the Carer having to give up work, or the missing salary of your charge, then you should apply for the necessary benefits. You will be entitled to Carer's Allowance if your partner is receiving Disability Living Allowance (DLA). All ostomates are entitled to DLA. Income support will also ensure you have a minimum income. You can receive both Carers Allowance and Income Support. Dependent upon age you may be entitled to Pension Credit or Attendance Allowance for your charge (In place of DLA – cut off age 65). Ask for a full benefits review to ensure you are receiving your maximum allowances as you may also be entitled to help with council tax and interest on your mortgage payments. For further information see; **www.direct.gov.uk**

For us, life changed on the 22rd March 2004 when, without any warning, my wife collapsed. From that date forward her health declined rapidly, she has been hospitalised many times, had countless blood transfusions, and a cocktail of medications. Her situation culminated in major surgery on On December 22nd. In August 2010, she had a second operation to replace her initial stoma, relocating it to the other side of her abdomen but this caused s stomal hernia and she is scheduled for additional surgery in 2011.

My first question to the doctors was, "What's wrong?" They just shook their collective heads "It could be..." they said, then gave a list of possible ailments but on one thing they all agreed, she was indeed a very sick lady. A fairly obvious fact to my mind given the number of tubes attached to her, pumping large quantities of various forms of antibiotics and other medication into her system. This was to be the beginning of what all carers experience: Endless hospital visits, the weariness and a full gamut of emotions - fear, loneliness, confusion, self-pity, anger, you name it, and like you, I have felt it.

In my situation, there were three possible outcomes:

- Elizabeth would not make it through this illness! I quickly disregarded this notion as something I would have to deal as and when.

- She would come home fit and well and we would pick up life where we left it. This was foolish, as the doctors had already told me that her symptoms had already caused a lot of permanent internal damage.

- That our lives would change, and we would work together to make the best of it.

Unwanted Baggage

Option three was the one I could live with and do something about. I'm a half-glass full sort of person, but now I felt as useful as an ashtray on a motorbike. I now had to do something, not just for my wife Elizabeth, but also for me. Yes, I discovered that it is perfectly fine to think about my own needs.

My first action was to clean the house, not just a lick and promise but to make every nook and cranny shine. It may seem foolish, but it was something positive I could do and would ensure a germ-free environment for my wife to return to. I then wrote to the bank and mortgage company to explain the situation, thus circumventing any financial problems that might arise. To their credit they responded within a few days, thanking me for informing them of the unfortunate situation and, given the circumstances, they were prepared to work with me if problems arose. I also contacted social services asking what help I could have if required. Theirs was also a positive reaction but they would need to know more about our needs when my wife came home.

Before her illness, my wife was the sort of person who seemed able to juggle six balls in the air while driving a motorbike around the wall of death, rarely taking even an aspirin. Elizabeth returned home after nearly four weeks in hospital and that is when our lives really changed. Even with the aid of crutches, she could barely walk across a room and had a prescription list of medications involving fifteen tablets, twice a day.

She had loved cooking but could no longer even pick up a pot or pan. We loved dancing and walking together through the fields of our small farm. Now it was up to me alone to care for the animals while she could not even walk outside unaided. There was still no diagnosis, no answers to all our questions.

During the next four years, we sold the farm and moved to a house more suited to my wife's needs. Social services installed a stair lift, bath lift and a variety of other aids. We replaced our sports car with a camper van so she could travel more comfortably (in a prone position). I dusted off and embellished my old cooking skills to provide tempting menus. More importantly, we began to learn how to get on with our lives despite the problems we now faced.

There were some answers to our questions, for some unknown reason Elizabeth's immune system had failed allowing a virus to attach itself to most of her joints. We were told that this virus had damaged or destroyed the thin membrane that lies between the muscle and skin at these points culminating in a diagnosis of Fibromyalgia, anaemia and hypoglycaemia. In August 2007, she suffered a grand mal seizure and if that was not enough, in December 2007, she underwent an emergency operation to remove her large bowel and had a bag fitted to her side. The resultant biopsy confirmed that she also had Crohn's disease.

While there is a great deal of very good advice on "caring", most of it appears to have been produced by "armchair" carers, who, like armchair footballers, have never actually played the game.

After six years of caring for my wife, I feel I have indeed played the game and have plenty of mud on my boots. I have learnt a few moves, tricks, and sometimes played

Unwanted Baggage

the blind side of the ref. not just to deal with my wife's problems but also my own.

I do not presume to say that our way of dealing with our situation is the right way because, providing it is medically safe and legal, then whatever way works for you is the right way. However, there are some real guidelines that we have found to be helpful:

Communication is vital!

Perhaps because we had both worked in areas where good communication skills were essential, talking to each other was, and remains, just one of the many joys of our relationship. For many people however, talking about their feelings is difficult. This is not a fault, just a simple fact. However, the more you understand about each other during these difficult times, the better it can help prevent mutual negative feelings such as isolation, anger and frustration. While it is perfectly natural to have these emotions, it is not good if these feelings are allowed to fester or turn in upon each other. If you find it difficult to talk about your feelings, then why not write notes to each other. This will give you time to explain how you feel about something that has happened which has upset you or about reactions that you do not understand.

For example:

- Statement: "I reached out and touched your arm, you pulled away, and it upset me."

- Answer, "Sorry, but my skin is so sensitive, it felt like sandpaper being dragged across it. I was not pulling my arm away from your touch, simply reacting to the pain at the time."

Colour cards are also a good idea in easing communication. You can produce these on a daily basis:

- Red "I'm not feeling very well and I'm in a bad mood."

- Yellow "Not feeling so bad but I might be a bit snappy."

- Green "Feeling pretty good can manage a hug."

Those uphill Emotions

You may have always been an upbeat and outgoing type or perhaps quiet and reserved –why try to change who you are. As your osto -"mate" may be very restricted in what they can now do, they may take out their anger and frustration out on you, the carer. It is said, "You often hurt the one you love." This is an unfortunate reaction and, while directed **to you**, is not necessarily directed **at you.** Nevertheless, it is still hurtful, and often feels unfair and undeserved. Think of it as the condition talking.

While a carer can walk away and work off these feelings your osto -"mate" cannot. Therefore, we have come up with the angry bag. My wife writes down all her anger on bits of paper, i.e. "I'm fed up of being stuck in the house." or "I wish I could do a bit of gardening.", whatever the mood dictates. She then screws these bits of paper into a ball and puts them all into a small bag. I then throw the bag into the rubbish. This does not take the problem away, but does help defuse the situation. Talking or writing notes to each other can help.

Perhaps guilt is the biggest problem to overcome. People often feel guilt even when they have no control over an event. It sometimes happens to survivors of terrible accidents or soldiers who survive when friends and colleagues are killed. Therefore, it is easy to understand that when someone becomes so ill that it drastically changes their lives and, more importantly, their way of thinking; it directly affects the lives of those people around them. The patient feels guilty and responsible for all the trouble they think they are causing and for the burden they believe they have become.

Guilt is like a great stone that hangs around my wife's neck. She did not choose to be ill, to suffer years of pain and immobility, yet the great stone is still there. So I asked a simple question: "If it was me lying in that bed, if it was me crying at night with the pain, if it was me that changed our life so much even though it was not my fault, would you not care for me as I do for you?". I know the answer really would be yes, and while the stone is still there, I hope it is lighter than before.

Information

In what seems a heartbeat, your world has been turned upside down. However, after a while it seems to settle into a routine. The upheaval slowly becomes the norm and a level of manageability develops. It is important not to become complacent. As the initial panic fades and you become more confident in dealing with this new way of life, remember there is the possibility that new and sudden developments may arise at any time.

Once we had an idea of the diagnosis, we decided on the path of enlightenment. We tried to find out all we could about the ailments. We talked to doctors, pharmacists, nurses, associations, and used the internet and the library. We found that knowledge is a key factor in helping deal with the situation and in anticipating sudden changes. Understanding your patient's illness to the best of your ability and being able to monitor the speed and manner in which they respond to their medication gives you a benchmark that you then can use to gauge their health level at any particular time.

We have simple tools such a digital thermometer, sugar level and blood pressure monitors that are all easy to use and provide immediate information. If a person's mobility is restricted, this can interfere with other bodily functions, such as digestion, kidney and bag problems, that can lead to pain, diarrhoea into the bag and severe bladder infections. Your osto -"mate" may be reluctant to complain about an additional problem or simply do not realise that one exists; but if **you** have established the norm, **you** can pick up on any changes quickly.

Mood, lack of appetite, high temperature, nausea and/or the time it takes for the medication to work are all early indicators that there could be an underlying problem. As most ostomates tend to take a cocktail of medication, do take advice as to which other simple forms of over-the-counter medication you can use to reduce temperature, relieve diarrhoea, nausea etc.

Unwanted Baggage

I would like to add a special note on the help you can get from your local social services department. Initially they will do an assessment. The Occupational Therapy Department will assess your needs for any equipment or alterations to your accommodation that might help you as a carer and your patient.

Following that The Adult Team or Children's Team will assign a case manager. He or She will conduct an assessment consisting of up to ten visits. They will talk to the GP, district nurse and other professionals involved in the care of you and the ostomate. The assessment will report on both your own needs as the Primary Carer and the Patient. I would like to mention Katie Derby and Michelle Raddie of Ceredigion Social Services. who gave us their help, care and support above and beyond anything we expected.

I have always advocated that carers should seek as much help and information as possible, so we took part in a social service carers and patient assessment. Don't panic it's not a test nor is there any pain, just simple one-on-one confidential chats with your caseworker and a simple questionnaire. Your caseworker will even help you complete the forms that ask such things as "Do you know your entitlements? "Do you know where else to get help?" and "Do you need other services that they think might be available to you?". While sometimes vilified by the media, Social Services help millions of families like ours every day.

As a carer, your own health and wellbeing is a very important factor, so respite, help with physical tasks and social care is all assessed. These assessments are not some form of means test and are voluntary, applying to both full and part time carers. You (the carer) have the opportunity to express your needs, what you might find difficult and where you might need help. Physical tasks, due to your own health or age, may have become a problem or a few hours of free time would be a great boost (recharging the batteries).

The resultant help could involve arranging physical additions to the house, equipment or counselling. It could also take the form of hands-on assistance or Direct Payments, an allowance to pay a friend or neighbour or even help finding an employee, to spend an hour or two with the person in you care, which is known as Social Care. Direct Payments can also cover Physical Care (washing/bathing etc. for your patient). The simple aim is to help you cope in difficult times when sometimes a little help can go a long way for you and the one you care for.

Finally, just because your partner is depressed does not mean that he or she always will be. They can't be forced into getting better, time alone is the greatest healer. When you truly care, time spent together is worth everything, no matter what the circumstances.

Carer's Contacts

Caring With Confidence – England Only
www.caringwithconfidence.net
Carrwood Park, Selby Road
Leeds LS15 4LG
Telephone: 0800 849 2349 (Carer Information Line)
Email: cwc.info@caringwithconfidence.net

Unwanted Baggage

Caring with Confidence is a free programme of flexible sessions for carers to help make a positive difference to their lives and that of the person they care for. Carers can get involved with Caring with Confidence in three ways – through <u>local group sessions </u>alongside other carers from their local community or from home using flexible <u>self-study workbooks </u>or <u>online sessions </u>designed to be completed at a pace to fit in with the demands on your time.

The programme is made up of several stand-alone <u>sessions</u> covering different topics that allow you to pick and choose, depending on your own caring situation.

Sessions look at things like practical aspects of day-to-day caring, communicating with others, financial and other resources and looking after your own health and wellbeing.

For carers attending local group sessions, they can also help with the cost of any alternative care required and travel to the venues. Caring with Confidence is completely free to any carer aged 18 and over in England.

Carers UK
<u>www.carersuk.org</u>
- nationwide
Telephone: 0808 808 7777
Carers UK is the voice of carers. Carers provide unpaid care by looking after an ill, frail or disabled family member, friend or partner. Carers give so much to society yet as a consequence of caring, they experience ill health, poverty and discrimination. Carers UK is an organisation of carers fighting to end this injustice.

Carers UK improves carers' lives by:

- campaigning for the changes that make a real difference for carers
- providing information and advice to carers about their rights and how to get support
- mobilising carers and supporters to influence decision-makers
- gathering hard evidence about what needs to change
- transforming the understanding of caring so that carers are valued and not discriminated against.

Crossroads Caring for Carers
www.crossroads.org.uk
Telephone : 0845 450 0350

Crossroads Caring for Carers has over 30 years experience of providing practical support services for carers and the people they are supporting. The key purpose of Crossroads Caring for Carers is to ensure that carers can have a break so services aim to be flexible and respond to individual situations. The services are of dual value - emotional support and a break for the carer, and a high-quality tailored service for the person they are supporting. Delivered through a network of local schemes in England, services may vary according to local need.

Every Crossroads Caring for Carers scheme is a member of Crossroads Association - the umbrella body for the network. The Association provides comprehensive policy and quality frameworks, as well as advice and guidance for local schemes and in addition works nationally with partners in the statutory and voluntary sectors to raise awareness of the needs of carers and contribute to policy development.

Family Carer Support Service (FCSS) - England only
www.hft.org.uk/carerssupport
Telephone: 0117 906 1751

The Family Carer Support Service would like all family carers and their learning disabled relatives to lead full, well supported lives. FCSS works to provide free services throughout England at individual, local, regional and national levels. They provide information and support to families through:

- personal contact by telephone, letter and email
- workshop courses in which we share knowledge, skills and support
- occasional conferences and seminars for family carers and/or professionals
- family Carer News Digests about policy, practice and carers issues
- developing other family focused materials and publications

- partnership working with other organisations, including the National Family Carer Network and the National Valuing Families Forum

Carers Direct
www.nhs.uk/carersdirect
Tel: 080880120202

Carers Direct is a practical and comprehensive information and advice service for Carers. You can call the helpline if you need help with your caring role and need to talk to someone about basically anything. The helpline advisors have resources to answer anything about assessments, benefits, direct payments, individual budgets, respite etc.

The helpline will also tell you how to complain if anything goes wrong with any of the services you use or put you in contact with your local authority of NHS services,. They are there to offer help when you most need it.

Carers Wales
www.carerswales.org
River House, Ynysbridge Court
Gwaelod y Garth
Cardiff CF15 9SS
Telephone: 029 2081 1370

Carers Wales is part of Carers UK. It works for a better deal for all carers in Wales. It is a policy, campaigning and information organisation.

Unwanted Baggage

In Wales, it maintains contact with carers through our membership and networks of branches and affiliates. It uses the experience of carers to:

Influence government policy through the National Assembly for Wales
Work to improve the services that affect the lives of carers at local level Inform carers of their rights and what help is available.
Campaign with others on UK wide issues such as benefits for carers.

Carers Scotland
www.carersscotland.org
The Cottage
21 Pearce Street
Glasgow G51 3UT
Telephone 08088087777

Carers Scotland is part of Carers UK. It works for a better deal for all carers in Scotland. .it is a policy, campaigning and information organisation.

Carers Scotland is working closely with the Scottish Government in developing a new strategy for unpaid carers in Scotland. This strategy will build on Care 21: the future of unpaid care in Scotland and set out plans to support carers for the next 10 years. The strategy group is made up of representatives of the Scottish Government, the Convention of Local Authorities in Scotland, carer's organisations, health and other statutory and voluntary sector organisations. A carer's reference group has been established to comment on progress and a carer from this group is represented on the main strategy steering group.

Supporting the work of the Strategy Group are a number of sub groups on key issues including breaks from caring, personalisation, training and personal development. A separate group has been established to take forward a strategy for young carers in Scotland that will form a distinct part of the overall strategy.

For more information on the strategy including minutes of meetings and progress to date, visit the dedicated section of the Scottish Government's site at
www.scotland.gov.uk/Topics/Health/care/Strategy

Carers Northern Ireland
www.carersni.org
58 Howard Street
Belfast BT1 6PJ
Telephone: 02890439843

Carers Northern Ireland is the voice of carers. Carers provide unpaid care by looking after an ill, frail or disabled family member, friend or partner. There are 185,000 carers in Northern Ireland.

Carers give so much to society yet because of caring, they experience ill health, poverty and discrimination. Carers Northern Ireland is an organisation of carers fighting to end this injustice. It will not stop, until people recognise the true value of carers' contribution to society and carers get the practical, financial and emotional support they need.

Chapter Twenty-three
Cooking for Carers
... Strangers to the kitchen?

By Philip Prosser

This chapter is dedicated to those who are unfamiliar with the process of cooking; perhaps believing you need a Degree to know how to make toast and that boiling an egg is in fact an act of God. Maybe that the kitchen is where the Food Fairies live a sort of magic grotto where you leave unprepared food and it mysteriously prepares itself into a meal.

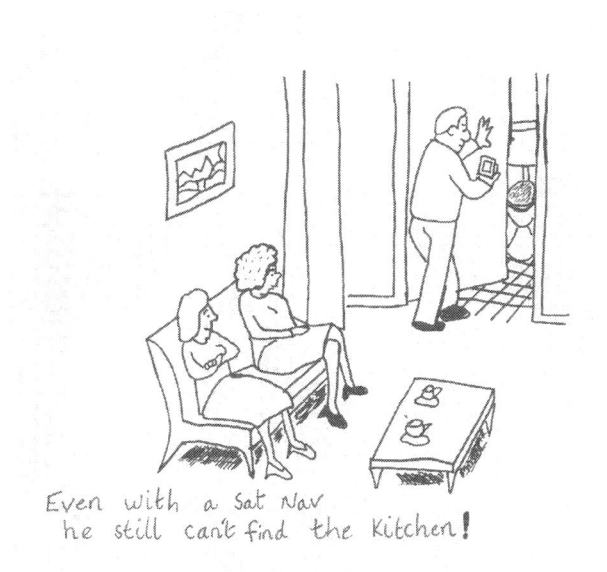

Even with a Sat Nav he still can't find the kitchen!

Take-away, ready meals and home delivery services are always available but they can be very expensive especially if you have other people depending on you (young children, elderly relatives etc.). In learning or improving your existing cooking skills, you may find that you get a taste for it (Pun intended), and move on from the simple meals to the gourmet stuff. Accepting the cooking challenge may also distract you for a short while from other problems you may have at this time.

If you have always been a passenger in a car and can't drive, you know that there are pedals on the floor of the car and there are levers and a round wheel but only some idea on how they all come together to make the car go. Tackle Cooking as you would driving, going from a former spectator enjoying the ride to getting behind the wheel. My first bit of advice to the Cooking Rookie is do not Panic! I am not going to ask you to fly a Jumbo Jet, simply to attempt to cook a few easily made meals. Cooking is a little knowledge mixed with some practice and a sprinkle of confidence.

Your first task will of course be to shop. In the past, you may have aimlessly pushed the shopping trolley around while the Master Chef of the household filled it with goodies while you moved trance-like up and down the aisles. Now you are on your own. It is just you, alone armed with your wits, and money against the SHOP. (Please note combat gear is not necessary just a pound coin for the trolley). Remember you will have a secret weapon: The shopping list.

Unwanted Baggage

The Shopping List.

Make a leap of faith here and trust me with the following basics. All will be revealed.

- 10 Large baking potatoes
- 3 large red Onions (Yes they do come in this colour)
- 6 large eggs
- 1 tin of corned beef,
- 2 packs of butter (1 for cooking and 1 for sandwiches if all else fails)
- 1 /12 litre bottle of basic olive oil (don't fall for the pricy stuff.
- 1 small bottle of brandy (a cheap 20cl size). This is for cooking but if all else fails....
- 1 bottle of mayonnaise
- 2 tins of sliced carrots
- 1 bag of grated cheese
- 1 lettuce – Cos or leafy (ask the staff!)
- 1 pack tomatoes
- 2 litres of milk
- 1 loaf of bread.
- Also get a potato peeler (This is not someone who comes to peal your spuds but a small tool)
- a food grater
- a pair of oven mitts or gloves
- 1 roll cling film
- 1 roll aluminium foil
- 1 apron – silly if possible

You may have these items already – but do you know where to find them?

If you want to look the part, you can buy an apron (Yes silly ones are OK) it does have the added advantage of keeping your clothes clean and covers all the hygiene aspects. Now, don't get distracted by the elevator music, shiny objects and the flashing lights. You do not need a forty- two inch flat screen TV just now! **Stick to the list,** then simply pay and leave
.

Home at last with a job well done; put all your goodies in the kitchen, the milk, butter and the tin of corned beef in the refrigerator then sit down have a break with a nice hot drink and take a look around. Remember that a kitchen is where you cook food not yourself. While it is not a battle zone, there will be very hot equipment and surfaces as well as hot liquids and sharp objects. Take your time, if you have a problem - turn everything off. Always use the oven gloves/mitts when handling hot equipment and always cut away from you when using a knife, although this is common sense, current 'elf 'n safety demands I say it.

For your first attempt, set aside some time when you are alone with no interruptions and plenty of room so if you blunder, just clean up and no one will know.

Most kitchens have a microwave oven. It looks like a television but has no pictures when you put it on, found it? Good. Now the basic variety has two controls one for power the other for time. (If it has any more dials, then I am afraid you will have to unearth the manual Aargh!). You need to turn the dial to high. Next, take two of your largest potatoes, give them a wash and jab them all over with a fork. Put the potatoes on any plate, (even paper will do – no metal or enamel ones please); wrap a piece

Unwanted Baggage

of cling film around the lot; then make a few small holes in the cling film to allow the steam to escape. Put this in the microwave and turn the time on to **8** minutes. When you shut the door, it will start. If a light comes on and you see the through the glass that your spuds are now slowly, almost romantically, moving around together then - congratulations, you on your way to your first jacket potatoes.

Don't open the Champagne just yet, this is only round one, you have to wait until the bell rings and the microwave stops. Open the door and, using your oven gloves/mitts, remove the plate and push a knife into your spuds - if knife passes through them easily the way they would if you were eating them, then they are cooked. Now remove the film, slice the potatoes open and put a pat of butter and sprinkle of grated cheese on top and put them back in the microwave for about a minute.

When the bell rings this time, it's all over, you have cooked yourself two cheese filled jacket potatoes! Well done! Remember your stoma patient must not eat the skins but they will enjoy the delicious centres especially because you have cooked them yourself. Potatoes and cheese provide the excellent protein that stoma patients need.

If you do not have a microwave, simply jab the spuds with a fork as before, wrap them in aluminium foil and put them in the oven on 200° C for about 45 minutes. Remove using an oven glove or tea towel and check with a knife, if they feel hard, then cook them for another 10 minutes or until our knife test works. When cooked, turn the oven off and close the door. Unwrap the foil, put your filling inside the spuds, rewrap and put them back in the oven for five minutes or so - the oven will still be warm enough to melt the filling. Remove, unwrap and eat.

There is a difference in the taste between the Micro-cooked and oven-baked potato as one is cooked in its own liquid while the other baked in a dry heat. If you want to keep them for later, let then cool, wrap in cling film or foil and put in the refrigerator until you want them. The normal rule with food is that you can heat it twice. Once, when it is cooked from raw and the second time to reheat it. (Providing the cooked food has been stored in the refrigerator for no more than two days.)

To store cooked food always make sure it's cold before you wrap or cover it and then place in a refrigerator at no more that 4 degrees or simply freeze
.

After your obvious success with the potatoes, you are ready to move on to your next sumptuous concoction. Put the kettle on. (Water heats quicker boiled in a kettle than in a saucepan on the hob.) Whilst it is boiling, locate a medium size saucepan. (i.e. a pot with a handle on one side and one that is big enough to put in four eggs). When the water has boiled, pour the contents into a saucepan (about 2" from the top). Turn a hotplate on to its highest setting and pop the pan on so that the water continues to boil. Use a spoon and put four eggs in the water. You want to see the little devil dancing about for about four minutes then, simply remove from heat and allow the water and eggs to cool down.

The difference between gas and electric is that you can turn off the gas and its heat stops immediately; electric cools down gradually. So, with an electric hob, always

Unwanted Baggage

remove a pot or pan, as it will continue to cook, even when turned off.

Once the eggs have cooled enough so that you can handle them easily, remove the shells (Great that they come ready wrapped); wash them under the tap to make sure there are no bits of shell left on them. Pop all the eggs into a bowl and mash with a fork. Add a little mayonnaise and mash again. You can add a pinch of salt and pepper to taste. After a few minutes, you will have egg mayonnaise sandwich filling. Cover and put in the fridge or make sandwiches to eat now. Another great stoma approved meal. This is just getting too easy isn't it?

Just when you thought I was a big softy, I am going to turn up the heat, literally!

Take two onions and a sharp knife – If you can't find a specific cooking knife, then a steak knife will do at a pinch. You should have a cutting or wooden board or you can use a flat clean ceramic or glass worktop for the next bit. The onion has two ends, the roots at one end and a pointy bit at the other, lay the onion on its side and cut both ends off. Discard the ends. This will leave you with two flat ends, stand the onion on one end and cut it down the middle from top to bottom.

You can see that the onion consists of rings - remove the outer ring (this will remove the skin do this with both sides and with both onions). Discard the skins and place each half face down on the surface, hold firmly and roughly cut from side to side so that you have a pile of semicircles. This does not have to be perfect, do take your time. TV chefs that you might have seen doing this at a hundred miles an hour have been practicing for years. You what a pile of onions, not fingers.

You now need a frying pan (The tennis racket shaped thing without holes) about 2 inches deep. Pour in a little olive oil and swish it around the pan so that there is a little on the sides and bottom. If you hold the pan to the light, you should see a film of t oil and that's all you need. Put in a large spoon (soup or dessert sized!) of butter and put on a low heat to slowly melt the two together.

When the oil and butter are mixed, turn up the heat a few notches (when you put the first bits of onion in there should be a nice sizzling noise).

Put at least one and a half of your onions into the pan, keep a little back, wrap it and put in the fridge for later. Now add a two spoons (same size as before), of water into the pan. Retrieve the Brandy. Open, fill up the cap and pour into pan. Pop a lid on the pan and let, as the professionals say the onions sweat. If you can't find a lid (as "other-halves" have a mysterious habit of hiding them), use aluminium foil as a cover. After a few minutes a stir your concoction. Your aim is to turn the crunchy onions, soft. If they are sticking to the pan, add a little more butter or a spoon of water and turn the heat down a little. Do this for about five minutes or until the onions are soft enough to break with your spoon, then remove from the heat but leave the lid on.

Locate the spuds and choose about 6-8 medium sized ones. Select a saucepan to fit with at least 3" to spare. Take your potato peeler by the handle. This looks a bit odd with a small handle an arch type piece of metal and a

Unwanted Baggage

thin piece of metal that connects the end of the top back to the handle (Bit like an axe saw). Now holding a spud in one hand pull the thin piece away from you over the spud and the skin should come off - the skin of the potato that is, not your skin. (I always do it towards, but the 'elf and safety lot say "away"!!) Once peeled, wash them and cut the potatoes into smaller pieces. Put the kettle back on, and when boiled, pour the water into the saucepan so that it covers the potatoes. Place the saucepan on the hob at a high heat and let it bubble for a few minutes. Turn the hotplate down and let it simmer for about 10-15 minutes. The potatoes will be cooked when you can push a knife through them like the jacket ones you did earlier.

While they are cooking open a two tins of carrots, pour away the brine in the cans. Open and empty the tin of corned beef you put in the fridge earlier. By putting it in the fridge, the meat inside the tin should be solid and easy to cut. Slice two thin pieces from the wide end, Wrap these in cling film or foil and return them to the fridge. When the potatoes are cooked, drain and separate into thirds, put a one third to cool in one bowl, another third into a similar bowl and return the rest into the empty pot.

Add the remaining large piece of corned beef, the onions and their juices from the frying pan into the large pot of potatoes and stir. Cover all the contents of the pot with water plus about 1" above. Leave the pan on a low heat so that the water looks as if it is simmering and cover. The corned beef will the slowly be absorbed into the mixture. After a ten minutes stir and then let it heat gently for a further ten minutes, stirring occasionally. Your meal is now ready to eat. You can also let this go cold and reheat again when all the contents have mixed. You can also freeze in a sealed container

You can then add a splash of milk, a spoonful of butter and the slices of the corned beef that you refrigerated earlier to one leftover third of the potatoes (in the bowl), and mash with a fork until it is all blended together, and then leave to cool. You now have a corned beef hash that you can fry or grill. Alternately, roll spoonfuls of this into balls with your hands, flattening them a little using the heel of our hand you have created a fritter (Well done you). You can fry these in a little hot oil in your frying pan, turning over as each side turns a browns slightly. You can also put the fritters on a lightly oiled metal tray in a hot oven (200°C), until brown. When cooked, serve the hash or fritters with a little chopped lettuce and tomato.

Cut the remaining piece of refrigerated raw onion into small pieces, chop up the remaining third of the cold potatoes and mix in the bowl. Add some mayonnaise and a teaspoon of vinegar for a rough potato salad. You can serve this with another sliced boiled egg, lettuce and tomatoes. Now have a rest, you made a stew, corn beef hash and a simple potato salad. You have some stuffed jacket potatoes and an egg mayonnaise for sandwiches.

When they pop up, cover with a little cheese, pop onto a metal tray and put under the grill until the cheese and melted and slightly browned. Eat and enjoy while warm.

Snack number two: Boil the kettle. When the water is boiled pour into a frying pan and put the pan on a high heat until you see streams of bubbles rising up, add a half teaspoon of vinegar Crack two eggs into the hot water

Unwanted Baggage

and put two pieces of bread in the toaster. The eggs will be nicely poached by the time the toast pops up. Butter the toast or not (to taste). Using one of those large spoons with holes in, fish out you the eggs. Let the water drain and pop an egg on each piece of toast, Poached egg on toast.

These may not be the most exciting of meals but they are filling, simple, cheap to buy and easy to prepare. I hope you try at least one or two of these suggestions. Cooking can be adventurous, therapeutic, productive and fun.

As a carer, I said that there would be changes; the glass should always be half-full, never half-empty.

Phil.

The Website
www.bowelmovement.co.uk
...The Future World of Unwanted baggage

The Book represents the "Harbour" of constants – of problems that will always occur.

The new website

www.thebowelmovement.co.uk

will be a flowing sea of change, bringing with each tide a flotsam and jetsam of new ideas to be salvaged and put to good use.

On the First tide, a new family will sail into port.

The Gastronauts

are a group of puppets who will brave the world on behalf of children everywhere. They will seek new young friends within the ostomate community to talk about problems and making the best of life with a stoma.

Other characters will sail in. There will certainly be a wealth of new products, ideas , reviews and stories for all ages.

Unwanted Baggage

Regular Competitions and discussions will keep you coming back for more!

Many useful ostomy-related products and the ostomy puppets may be purchased from the "Quayside" shop with a percentage of profit being donated to specific ostomy charities.

A visiting Chef will advise on existing new, inexpensive easy recipes. These can be found on the on the Carer's Corner where you can also find support information.

You are far from being alone. The Forum, open to all, will give you the opportunity to air your problems, solutions, ideas and thoughts.

We look forward to making your acquaintance online and ask your help in developing the site into an interesting, amusing, informative, innovative, exciting new Ostomate World.

Remember, if you ever see someone without a smile, give them one of yours.

Stoma Stuff!

Everything Else

websites and other useful information

The following is a listing of other information and websites that you might find useful or informative.

Abelize
www.ableize.com/index.php

This is the UK and Ireland's largest and most viewed resource of disability mobility and special needs. On this site, you can find disabled products, services, sports and holidays also the largest collection of disabled clubs, groups and charities in the UK. All this plus children's and childcare, education, wheelchairs and vehicles plus mobility, walking, daily living and bathing aids.

Ableize is owned and run by disabled people and has disability covered.

Accessatlast
www.accessatlast.com

This is a Directory of hotels with accessible toilets and other accessible features around the UK. Contains reviews from visitors.

Accessible Travel
www.accessibletravel.co.uk

This is a great world of accessible holidays and travel for wheelchair users, slow walkers, mature travellers their families and friends.

Action for Sick children
www.actionforsickchildren.org

This is an excellent support and advice site for parents and carers of children with chronic health conditions. There are some excellent publications and good advice on dealing with the NHS in relation to services for sick children and their parents.

All About Bowel Surgery
www.allaboutbowelsurgery.com

This is what it says on the label! A general information site run by the bag manufacturer Welland –While it does not go into enough detail in some areas, interestingly, it contains on cultural diversity affects surgery.

All Go Here
www.everybody.co.uk

This website provides information on hotels, airlines and other services that can be used by anyone, listing only mainstream hotels, and not those targeted towards only people with disabilities.

BOSS - Bristol Ostomists Self Support Group
www.ostomweb.org.uk

Bristol Ostomists regularly hold Saturday afternoon meetings including one-to-one presentations, counselling and discussion time.

Bladder & Bowel foundation
www.bladderandbowelfoundation.org

Telephone: 0845345533255
The Bladder and Bowel Foundation's website provides a great deal of information for anyone with bladder or bowel related problems. Their on-line library is extensive and contains many in-depth studies. From Pelvic Floor exercises to overactive bladders. Nocturia or nocturnal enuresis
? Discussions on health bowels to a range of incontinence products. Excellent links and support information. Highly Recommended.

BLISS
Special care baby
www.bliss.org.uk
Telephone: 05006181140

Bliss, the special care baby charity, provides vital support and care to premature and sick babies across the UK. Founded 30 years ago, they offer guidance and information at a critical time in families' lives. They also fund ground-breaking research and campaign for babies to receive the best possible level of care regardless of when and where they are born.

As a number of premature babies are born with bladder and bowel problems, this is a wonderful support organisation for those with newborns with problems.

British Council of Disabled People
www.bcodp.org.uk

The UK's national organisation of the worldwide **Disabled People's Movement -** promoting their full equality and participation in society.

British Society of Gastroenterology
www.bsg.org.uk

The British Society of Gastroenterology (BSG) exists to maintain and promote high standards of patient care in gastroenterology and to enhance the capacity of its members to discover and apply new knowledge to benefit patients with digestive disorders. Members include physicians, surgeons, pathologists, radiologists, scientists, nurses, dieticians, and others.
The site includes good information for all gastro patients including latest medical treatments and links to other professional medical sites.

C3Life
www.c3life.com

Note: This site is supported by the manufacturer Hollister.

C3Life.com is an online international ostomy community website; the majority of members are from the US. It allows people with an ostomy to contribute, interact and get involved and share experiences. Useful information sheets but, as it is run by a manufacturer, promotes its own products.

Calvert Trust
www.calvert-trust.org.uk

The Calvert Trust specialises in outdoor activities for disabled people, providing the professional expertise to expand and improve the range of activities available to people with disabilities

Child Growth Foundation
www.childgrowthfoundation.org

This site contains information of benefit to parents with a child who has a diagnosed or suspected growth problem, to people who have a growth problem and their families, and to people and medical professionals with an interest. As Crohn's disease can affect young children and adolescent growth, this site has some valuable links.

Colon Surgery Information
www.colonsurgeryinfo.com

It is important to know that there are effective treatment options for colon disease, such as minimally invasive surgery. Here you will find important information about diseases of the colon and their treatment options. Just spending a little time now to learn more about treatment options can make a big difference later. It is a US site, but has relevant, useful information for all patients.

Colostomy Association:
www.colostomyassociation.org.uk

The UK's national colostomates organisation. (See references throughout the book). It organises groups, newsletter etc. **Highly recommended.**

Connexions Direct
www.connexions-direct.com

Connexions Direct can help you with information and advice on issues relating to health, housing, relationships with families and friends, careers and learning options, as well as activities you can get involved in.

Council for Disabled Children
www.ncb.org.uk

The CDC provides a national forum for the development of policy and practical issues relating to service provision and support for children and young people with disabilities and special educational needs.

Crohn's and Colitis UK
www.crohnsandcolitisuk.org.uk
www.nacc.org.uk

Crohn's and Colitis UK (formerly known as the National Association of Colitis and Crohn's, its name change was in April 2010).

This is one of the most useful associations for IBS in the UK providing fact sheets on every topic and running a superb helpline and many other member services. Seventy-six local groups throughout the UK are there to welcome new members and hold regular events with medical and specialist speakers and simple get together meetings to compare notes.

I have referred to them many times in the text and they are **highly recommended.**

Crohn's Zone
www.crohnszone.org

Excellent support website for Crohn's and Colitis – They have an amusing forum, discussions on many aspects of Crohn's and ostomates. Silly products and lots of information. **Really good** blog spot.:

Chronic Pain Support
www.chronicpainsupport.org

Many people with ostomies have accompanying chronic pain. The primary goal at the Chronic Pain Support Group (CPSG) is to provide a safe Internet environment where those living in pain can get the support they need. Its message board and chat rooms are the primary sources of support CPSG believes that anyone in pain deserves to be treated with dignity by friends, family and the medical community without fear of being seen as malingering or a drug seeker. A critical component to the treatment of pain is support. Without adequate support, pain patients soon fall into despair. This organisation strives to provide support that will give hope for a better tomorrow.

Computers For The Disabled
www.cftd.co.uk/cftd.htm

This organisation provides quality recycled PC's & new parts supplied to the Disabled, the housebound, disabled centres & home users by our Non-profit organisation

DART
www.dart.org.uk

Includes information on transport issues such as Dial-a-Rides, accessible bus routes, tubes, Freedom Passes and the Blue Badge Scheme

Department for Transport Mobility and Inclusion Unit
www.dft.gov.uk/transportforyou/access

The Government's Quality Protect Programme is a key part of its strategy to prevent social exclusion. This Department of Health site contains information about the QPP for disabled children, such as news, policy developments, and links to relevant organisations.

DIAL UK
www.dialuk.info

The national organisation for the DIAL Network of 160 local disability advice centres ran by and for disabled people

Directgov
www.direct.gov.uk

Information for disabled people in areas such as employment, health and education. There is also advice on independent living, leisure, financial support and rights. General government advice site as well.

Disability Alliance
www.disabilityalliance.org

Publisher of the Disability Rights Handbook, the DA is regarded as the leading authority on social security benefit for disabled people

Disabled Gear
www.disabledgear.com

DisabledGear.com is the **FREE,** clear and totally user-friendly FREE-Ads website for buying and selling second hand disability equipment. It is designed to make the whole process painless. Its creator – a paralysed wheelchair user – wanted:

- classifieds to be free, so people use them, and the system works better for everyone: buyers have choice & sellers have buyers.

- to simplify buying and selling disability equipment, too often a frustrating and expensive business.

- a clear and attractive website that is easy to use and navigate around.

- one easy place for anyone with any disability to buy and sell second hand equipment.

Sellers register their details that allow the "search by distance" feature to work, and listing is a simple systematic process. Another safe feature of registration is that sellers can choose whether to show or hide private contact details or not, as potential buyers can make initial email contact through the site.

Buyers do not need to register, as they can browse freely, but must do so if they want the same "search by distance" feature to work. DisabledGear.com has a strict Privacy Policy so that private details are not abused.

A New Products section is in the pipeline, selling well designed and produced items. They are committed to cutting out the middle-men and therefore some of the unreasonable mark-ups.

Disabled Go
www.wdco.org/site/DisabledGo/index.htm

Provides guides to goods and services for disabled people, their carers, family and friends, it also aims to break down barriers to inclusion in the community.

Disabled Living Foundation
www.dlf.org.uk
380 384 Harrow Road
London
W9 2HU
Tel: 0845 1309177

Disabled Living Foundation provides free, impartial advice about all types of equipment for disabled adults, disabled children, older people, their carers and families. From stair lifts to walk-in baths, jar openers to tap turners, bath seats to walking sticks, wheelchairs to scooters, hoists to beds, the DLF can help you find solutions that enable you to stay active and independent life.

Find A&E/Dentist/GP
nhsdirect.nhs.ukif

If you are caught out, taken ill while travelling, then, using your mobile phone you can text for the details of the nearest A&E, GP or dentist. Simply text the name (i.e. GP) of the service you require to **61121** or for details contact the website.

Foundations/Care and Repair
www.foundations.uk.com
England
For help with repairs/painting etc. for disabled and people on income support or pension credit.

For Wales:
Care & Repair Cymru
029 20576 286
www.careandrepair.org.uk

For Scotland:
Care & Repair Forum Scotland
0141 221 9879
www.careandrepairscotland.co.uk

For Northern Ireland:
Fold Housing Association
02890 428314
www.foldgroup.co.uk

Home improvement agencies assist vulnerable homeowners and private sector tenants who are older, disabled, chronically sick or on a low income to repair, improve, maintain or adapt their homes. They are local, not-for-profit organisations.

Every home improvement agency provides a range of services depending on the needs of the local community. Their services can include some or all of the following.

- Providing a list of reliable local builders and contractors

- Visiting you at home to give advice about any problems you have with the condition of your home

- Setting out your housing options and helping you decide which is best for you

- Helping you obtain other local support services

- Checking whether you are entitled to any financial help (for example, disability benefits, or money to help you repair or adapt your home)

- Helping with any work you decide to have carried out on your home. For example, drawing up plans, getting estimates and liaising with others involved in the work, such as council grants officers and occupational therapists

- Additional services such as a handyperson services, to carry out small jobs around your home, help with gardening, or coming home from hospital

- Helping to make your home more energy-efficient.

Gay Ostomates Organisation
www.gayostomates.org

While this UK based website is aimed at gay ostomates worldwide, there is lots of general information for all ostomates.

The aim of this website is to provide news about events, products, health information in a friendly format and the chance to email each other and possibly meet up with the hope that life can be improved for many of us who often feel very isolated at times. Great contact site for the gay community.

Gay & Lesbian Ostomates of America
www.glo-uoa.org

Good all round site for information pertaining to gay and lesbians ostomates. The site also contains a lot of information for ostomates in general.

The Gut Trust
www.theguttrust.org

Unit 5
53 Mowbray Street
Sheffield
S3 8EN
Tel: 0114 272 3253

The Gut Trust is the national charity for people with Irritable Bowel Syndrome in the United Kingdom. It supports people who are coping day to day with IBS; a condition that is misunderstood, often stigmatised and which can chronically affect your everyday life.

Its support is in several ways. For members, it offers a telephone helpline staffed by medical and nursing specialists and on-line medical advice and consultation, factsheets on all aspects of IBS, online support, "can't wait "cards and "travel cards" to facilitate access to toilets at home and abroad, a quarterly magazine. Its interactive and frequently updated website includes a unique, fully comprehensive **Self Management Programme** to help live life to the full with IBS. **Highly Recommended**

Healthy socks
www.silversock.co.uk

Silver is recognised in the medical community as a very effective antimicrobial agent, proven to kill over 400 different types of bacteria. The X-Static Silver fibres use pure silver to inhibit the growth of odour-causing bacteria and fungi in the socks. Bacteria are only one source of foot odour. Ammonia and denatured proteins are also significant causes of odour in hosiery products.
Carnation Silversocks neutralise ammonia and denatured proteins because both bind readily to silver resulting in instant odour reduction. X-Static Silver eliminates 99.9% of bacteria in less than one hour of exposure. These socks are recommended for postoperative recovery (£5.99 pair).

IBD –UK
www.ibduk.com

This is an international blog site with wonderful utube videos from patients, and doctors, including one of the international experts on Crohn's disease, Dr Bill Sandborn from the Mayo Clinic. Updated and well maintained. **Warning:** The website also contains many advertisements containing "miracle cures" ergo **Treat with caution and a large pinch of salt!.**

Ileostomy Association of Great Britain:
www.the-ia.org

See all the references to this in the book. This is the only national UK organisation for all ileostomates. Organises groups, produces a Newsletter etc. **Highly Recommended**.

Inside Out Stoma Support Group
www.iossg.org.uk

Inside Out Stoma Support Group was set up in November 1999 and a few years later was incorporated with St Marks Hospital Foundation to provide continuing support, reassurance and practical information to anyone who may be about to have or who has already had one of the above stomas. It also provides support to their families and carers before, during and after surgery. They hold coffee mornings every two weeks, (see dates & details on the next page), its a place where you can let your hair down and talk to others who are going or gone through similar problems and learn how to resolve them. All ostomists are welcome as is their partners, family members and carers.

International Ostomy Association
www.ostomyinternational.org

The IOA is the association of all global Ostomy associations. It is committed to the improvement of the quality of life of Ostomates and those with related surgeries, worldwide. It provides to its member associations, information and management guidelines, helps to form new Ostomy associations, and advocates on all related matters and policies. It is organised to grow and develop while remaining independent and financially viable.

This site is an excellent resource for all ostomates and urostomates.

J Pouch Group
www.j-pouch.org

This site contains really useful information and contacts for people with a J-Pouch

The Kingston Trust
secretary@ktrust.org.uk

PO Box 6457
Basingstoke
Hants
RG24 8LG
01256 352320

The Kingston Trust is a registered charity whose aim is to provide assistance for elderly ileostomists experiencing financial hardship. They offer grants a a one-off payment for a specific need (i.e. washing machine, convalescent beak etc) or payments at regular intervals to supplement income.

Applications for any purpose will be considered. Routine payments are reviewed annually. Application forms can be obtained from the secretary.

M D Junction
www.mdjunction.com

This is a collection of support groups worldwide for all illnesses (including all IBD and urology illnesses).
MDJunction is an active centre for Online Support Groups and provides a place where thousands of patients meet every day to discuss their feelings, questions and hopes with like-minded friends. Free to join.

Macmillan Cancer Support
www.macmillan.org.uk

This charity provides practical, medical and financial support for people affected by cancer. This is a wonderful

Mobility Information Service
www.mis.org.uk
Unit B1 Greenwood Court
Carmel Drive
Shrewsbury
Shropshire
SY1 3TB
Tel: 01743 463072

MIS provides neutral advice on buying a car, scooter or other mobility aid. It also offers information on suppliers and on whom to contact for adaptations to vehicles. It provides guidance on your legal rights as a mobility road user; and general advice on tax, parking badges and other benefits.

Motability
www.motability.co.uk
Goodman House
Station Approach
Harlow
Essex CM29 2ET
Tel: 0845.456 4566

This is the official website of the Motability scheme. To lease a car from Motability, you must be receiving either:

- Higher Rate Mobility Component (HRMC) of the Disability Living Allowance (DLA) or,

- War Pensioners' Mobility Supplement (WPMS)

If you choose to lease a car through Motability's Contract Hire scheme, you must have at least 12 months' award length remaining. For customers choosing to buy a car with a Hire Purchase agreement, you will need to be receiving the allowance for the full length of your agreement

Mobility Trust
www.mobilitytrust.org.uk
17B Reading Road
Pangbourne
Reading
Berks
RG17 0NE
Tel: 0118 984 2588

The Mobility Trust will provide mobility equipment including the first year's insurance. The trust will consider anyone who has a disability. If you are not eligible for help from any other organisation, please write a letter explaining your circumstances to the trust.

National Advisory Service for Parents of Children with a Stoma

NASPCS

51 Anderson Drive
Valley View Park
Darvel
Aryshire
Tel: 01560 322024

Note: The contact is John Malcolm (Chairman), who works from home office hrs are 9-5. **The website www.naspcs.co.uk is not yet live.**

The NASPCS provides a contact and information service for parents on the practical day-to-day management of all aspects of coping with a child with a colostomy, ileostomy or urostomy.

They also try to give advice on the incontinence often encountered with bowel and bladder problems. Charity operated from home address. Do not hesitate to call for information or advice.

Need A Loo?

www.needaloo.org

The aim of Need A Loo is to list all the publicly accessible disabled toilet facilities in the United Kingdom (or anywhere else!), with maps showing locations.

To get started, just click on a country's name to go to that country's index.

Neuronal Intestinal Dysplasia /STC NiDKiDS
www.pcaa.org.au/new_page_3.htm

NiDKiDS is the only website that provides information and support to families, medical and allied health practitioners from all over the world that **support children and young people diagnosed with the bowel and bladder conditions**: Neuronal Intestinal Dysplasia (NID) more commonly known as Slow Transit Constipation (STC).

They produce a series of fact sheets that provides comprehensive information about assessment, diagnosis and treatment options for patients and their families. Whilst this information has been provided by PCAA under the guidance of the Paediatric Continence Advisory Council, the information is not intended to replace your physician's advice.

Ostomy Land
www.ostomyland.com

Unwanted Baggage

International ostomy support site, contains useful facts and links. Sponsored by the UOAA (United ostomy association of America).

Patients Association
For England
www.patients-association.com

(Also general UK-wide information)
For SCOTLAND
Your local NHS board will also be able to give you information on help from an independent advocate if you need help making your complaint. For further information about the NHS in Scotland:

www.show.scot.nhs.uk
www.hris.org.uk
(for health rights information only)

For WALES
Community Health Councils exist to offer help and advice to patients and your local Council may be found at : **www.patienthelp.wales.nhs.uk**

Each CHC has a Complaints Advocacy Service to assist with individual complaints.

For further information about the NHS in Wales:
www.wales.nhs.uk

For NORTHERN IRELAND
Health and Social Services Councils exist to offer help

and advice. For further information about the NHS in Northern Ireland: **www.hsni.net**

The Patients Association is an independent charity that highlights the concerns and needs of patients. It works with Government and a broad range of individuals and organisations to develop better, and more responsive, health services.

The Patients Association advocates for greater and more equitable access to high-quality, accurate and independent information for patients. Its aim is to reduce health inequalities by helping patients to be better informed and by campaigning for patients to have the right to be involved in decision-making.

Its role is to help provide patients with the information that is difficult to access; the information that is often hidden away by vested interest but is their legal right to know.

In the campaign to ensure patients are better informed, It has a range of patient guides and advice booklets .

Patients with Immune Deficiencies
www.pia.org.uk

The PiA is the only registered charity dedicated to supporting and helping children and adults with Primary Immunodeficiencies in the UK. They provide information for the newly diagnosed and the not so newly diagnosed in the form of newsletters, leaflets and an informative website. Through patient days and other PiA events, you will have the opportunity to meet up with others

Unwanted Baggage

who have similar rare conditions to your own, and share personal experiences.

They also organise holiday breaks for children and young people with primary immunodeficiencies, giving them the chance to get away and have fun. They can help you with information packs for children with primary immunodeficiencies who are starting school or college, and we can advise you on travel insurance and holiday planning.

There is no charge for membership, simply email your information to joimup@pia.org.uk

PSC – What is that?
www.psc-support.demon.co.uk

About 75% of PSC sufferers also have Ulcerative Colitis (UC). PSC stands for Primary Sclerosing Cholangitis, a no known cause, no known cure chronic and progressive disease of the bile ducts. The problem is inflammation of the bile ducts, both intra- and extra hepatic, resulting in scarring and narrowing of the ducts and limiting bile flow to the duodenum and often flowing back into the liver and killing off the liver cells.

Typical symptoms include: right upper quadrant pain or discomfort, severe itching, fatigue, together with the well known UC conditions. Diagnosis is not always easy, and many patients go undiagnosed primarily because of lack of knowledge or understanding of the condition by clinicians. Symptoms can be intermittent but then progress to a point where a liver transplant is the result.

Liver Function Tests (LFTs), MRCP (a specific abdomen-related MRI) or the endoscopic investigation known as ERCP are methods used to detect the disease.

RADAR
Royal Association For Disability and Rehabilitation
www.radar.org.uk
12 City Forum,
250 City Road,
London EC1V 8AF
Tel: 0171 250 3222
Best know to ostomates for its **National Toilet Key Scheme** that provides universal keys to disabled toilets nationwide, RADAR is a fantastic source of anything connected with the world of disability of any kind.

RADAR is also a resource for all advocacy issues and is currently actively campaigning against the new DLA medical examinations.

Regard
National Organisation of Disabled Lesbians, Gay Men, Bisexuals & Transgender People

Unit 2J Leroy House
436 Essex Road
Islington
London
N1 3QP
Tel: 020 7688 411

Regard was founded in 1989. Its aim is to raise awareness of disability issues within the Lesbian, Gay, Bisexual and Transgendered (LGBT) communities, and to raise awareness of sexuality issues within the disability communities. It also works to combat social isolation amongst our membership, and to campaign on issues specifically affecting disabled LGBT people.

Regard is an organisation that is run by the membership for the membership. They welcome membership applications from all those defining themselves as Disabled or chronically ill Lesbians, Gay Men, Bisexuals and Transgendered People, as well as from our friends and supporters. Membership is free.

Run – Pee!
www.runpee.com

This is not actually a vulgar website as the title suggests – it is however, of great use to those IBD patients who enjoy visits to the cinema or watching films on television channels without advertising.

It advises on the best places in new and even classic release movies to "skip to the loo". If you are connected to the web by mobile phone and have to make an unscheduled "dash", it will also text you the bits of the movie you have missed during your short excursion.

Not to be scoffed at for those who hate missing a vital part - or even worse - the ending!

United Ostomy Association of America
www.uoaa.org

The United Ostomy Associations of America, Inc. (UOAA) is a US based network for bowel and urinary diversion support groups in the United States. Its goal is to provide a non-profit association that will serve to unify and strengthen its member support groups, which are organized for the benefit of people who have, or will have intestinal or urinary diversions and their caregivers. While its website contains interesting information and how US ostomates cope with their healthcare problems. It has links to US suppliers, many of whom will export. It also provides an insight into the US view on ostomies. Worth checking out.

Urostomy Association
www.urostomy association.org.uk

This great organisation provides support for all UK urostomates. The site has loads of Information, the association runs national groups and has an excellent newsletter. Highly recommended.

The World Council of Enterostomal Therapists Education Committee
www.wcetn.org
UK Contact: Mrs B Borwell, - Stomatherapist,
Salisbury District Hospital,
Odstock Salisbury
Wiltshire SP2 8BJ
Tel: 0114 272 3253

A global organisation for colorectal nurses. This is the UK contact point for all nurses interested in joining. The Association provides all the latest information on all aspects of enterostomal care. Meetings and conferences are held worldwide.

That's all folks!
See you on the website with more stoma stuff!
www.thebowelmovement.co.uk

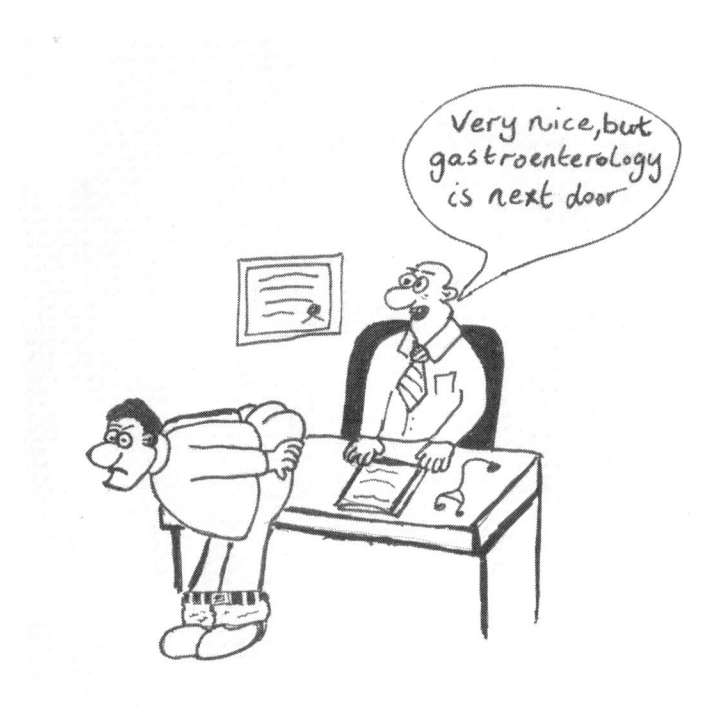

THE END